Serena Chellini

COMPENDIUM OF TRADITIONAL CHINESE MEDICINE

Youcanprint *Self-Publishing*

Title | Compendium of Traditional Chinese Medicine
Author | Serena Chellini
Cover photograph by the author Translation by Iolanda Foschetti

ISBN | 978-88-92610-13-2

Youcanprint Self-Publishing
Via Roma, 73 - 73039 Tricase (LE) - Italy
www.youcanprint.it
info@youcanprint.it
Facebook: facebook.com/youcanprint.it
Twitter: twitter.com/youcanprintit

I was delighted to be entrusted with the task of translating Serena's book on Traditional Chinese Medicine because, as a Shiatsu therapist and translator, I looked forward to working on a subject dear to my heart and hoped I would learn more about the subject as I translated.

I was not disappointed; it is a book full of interesting facts and areas of study that are not often found together. As Serena says in her introduction, this book is a collection of notes from years of seminars and courses and it introduces topics that are very remarkable and inspiring.

Each chapter has precious gems of information; the chapter on The Extraordinary Organs is particularly interesting and the many pages on the Extraordinary Vessels, their points and uses, is especially fascinating. There are lots of useful suggestions and snippets of information that have helped clarify many things that previously had never been very clear to me.

It is a very readable book. It can be read from start to finish or flicked through and the chapters read in any order. The layout is inviting too; the print is clear and the pages not overcrowded.

I also had the pleasure of meeting Serena Chellini when we spent a few days together at her home in Tuscany going through the translation.

She is a peaceful, gentle woman and her Shen radiates from her eyes and warmed my soul.

Iolanda Foschetti

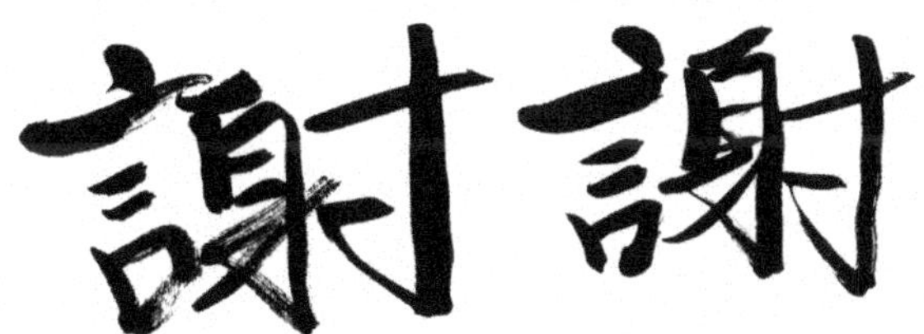

PREFACE

Initially I began to write this compendium for my own personal use so that I could have all the information at my fingertips, the knowledge I had acquired through more than ten years of study, seminars and practice.

From the start, Traditional Chinese Medicine and Shiatsu have captured my curiosity and with great passion, I have continuously strived to deepen my knowledge.

My aim is to provide basic and important information about TCM, which can be easily and quickly consulted.

I realize that certain topics cannot perhaps be completely comprehensive, but for any in depth facts, techniques and maps, I recommend looking at the existing specific texts available.

In all these years of practice, these 'notes' have been very helpful to me and I hope with all my heart that they can be useful to all those committed to travelling along this same evolutionary path.

May everyone find the road to self-realization and may their knowledge benefit others.

Enjoy this book and all the best in your work!

Serena Chellini

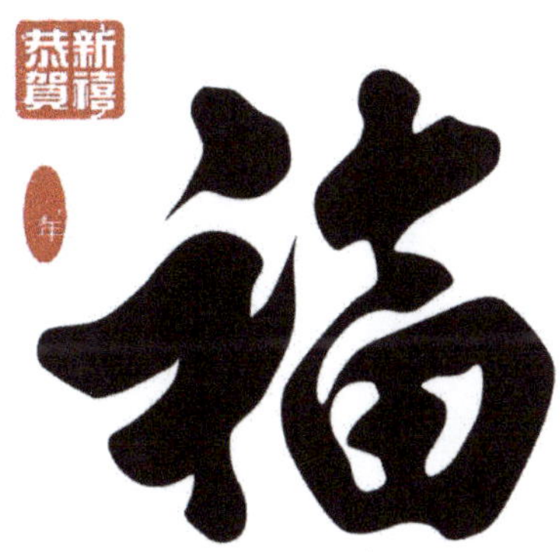

Acknowledgements

Yeshi Dhonden, the first person to show me how to work with love and passion

My parents

Massimo, my husband and life partner

My Masters and teachers

All my patients

Life, the greatest Teacher

And all of you who read this

May joy, health and prosperity fill each and every existence.

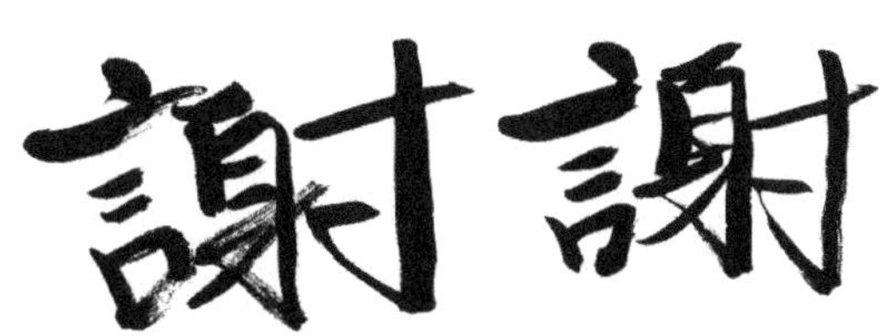

"In the pursuit of learning,
everyday something is acquired.
In the pursuit of Tao,
everyday something is dropped.
"Less and less is done
Until non-action is achieved.
When nothing is done,
nothing is left undone.

The world is ruled by letting things take their course.
It cannot be ruled by interfering."

Lao Tzu 'Tao Te Ching'

ABBREVIATIONS

HT	Heart
LV	Liver
LI	Large Intestine
SI	Small Intestine
SP	Spleen
PC	Pericardium
LU	Lungs
KD	Kidney
ST	Stomach
TB	Triple Burner
BL	Bladder
GB	Gall Bladder
CV	Conception Vessel (Ren Mai)
GV	Governing Vessel (Du Mai

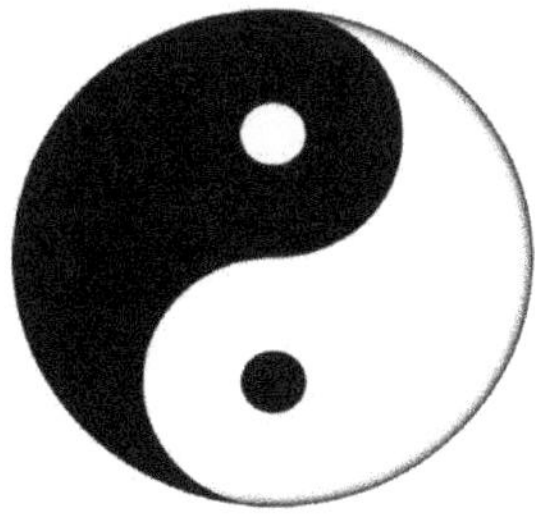

YIN – YANG

Opposing but complementary qualities.

Interdependent: one cannot exist without the other.

A two-stage process of change and transformation of all natural phenomena.

Each contains the root of the other.

Yang is external and protects, while Yin is internal and nourishes.

YIN is receptivity, the state of inertia and potential energy, the deep, dark and mysterious side. It is symbolized by the element Water for its natural tendency to flow downwards and to adapt to any shape and container, and also by the element Earth, that sustains and nourishes.

The Female Principle.

YANG is activity, action, the expression of potential energy, brightness, superficial, visible. It is symbolized by the element Fire for its natural tendency to move incessantly upwards, for its lightness and instability.

The Male Principle.

The **<u>Yang Meridians</u>** can be used to strengthen the Yang, to defend against external pathogenic factors, and to eliminate them when they have already invaded the body.

The **<u>Yin Meridians</u>** can be used to tonify the Yin.

All the Yang Meridians start or end on the head. Yang energy tends to rise and, in pathological situations, can cause the face and eyes to become red (Heat or Fire rising). The head is often affected by Yang pathogenic factors such as Wind and Summer Heat. The points on the head can also be used to increase Yang energy.

The chest and abdomen, being Yin, are easily affected by Yin pathogenic factors, such as Cold and Dampness.
The area above the navel (Yang) is easily affected by Yang pathogenic factors, such as Wind, whilst the area below the navel (Yin) is affected by Yin factors such as Dampness.

<u>The Fu Organs are Yang:</u> they transform and digest food, expelling impure residues; they communicate with the external world.

<u>The Zang Organs are Yin:</u> they accumulate the pure essences produced through the transformation process carried out by the Viscera, namely Qi, Blood, Body Fluids and Jing.

However, every organ has within it both a Yin and Yang aspect.
The structure of the actual organ, and the vital substances contained within, reflect the Yin aspect, while the functional activity of the organ reflects the Yang.

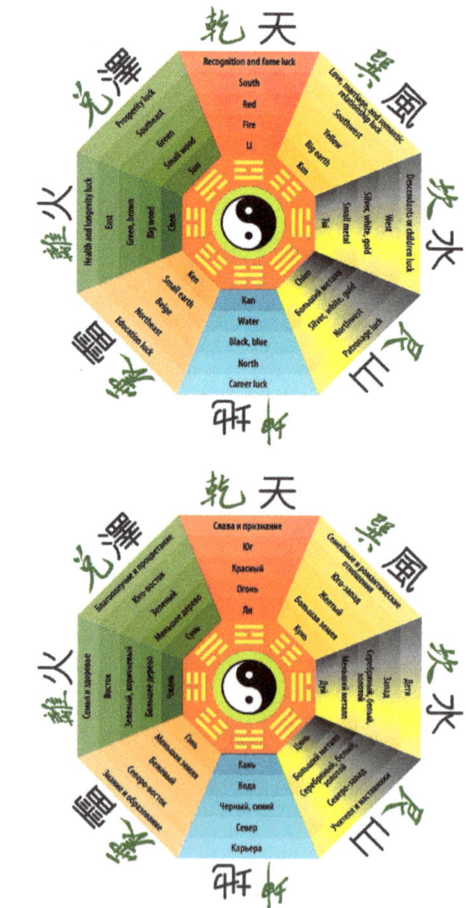

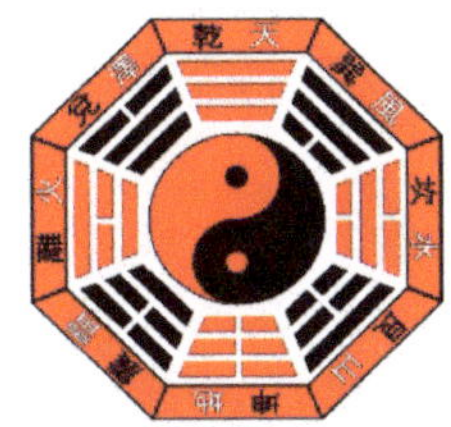

YANG	**YIN**
Day	Night
Brightness	Darkness
Summer	Winter
South	North
Outside	Inside
Sun	Moon
Heaven	Earth
Circle	Square
Activity	Rest
Movement	Receptiveness
Time	Space
Above	Below
Expansion	Contraction
Extroversion	Introversion
Energy	Matter
Light	Heavy
Male	Female
Rationality	Intuition
Rising	Descending
Fire	Water
Hot	Cold
Function	Structure
Viscera	Organs
Agitation	Tranquillity
Dry	Wet
Hard	Soft
Fast	Slow
Odd	Even

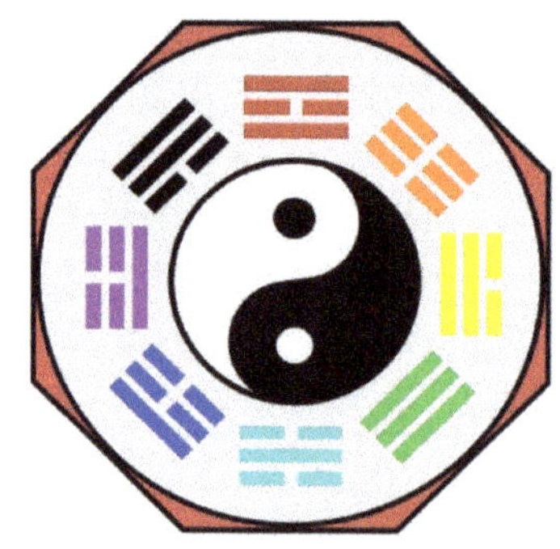

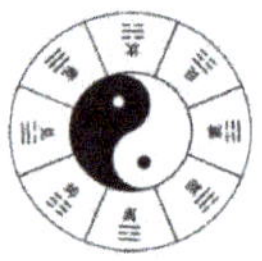 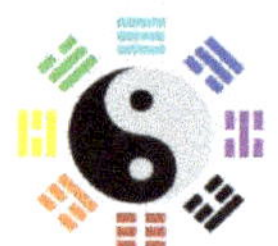 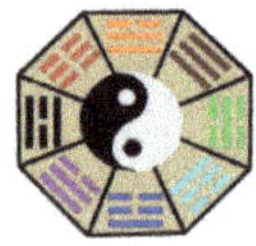

MAIN PATHOLOGICAL MANIFESTATIONS

<u>YANG</u>	<u>YIN</u>
Acute, recent illness	Chronic illness
Rapid onset	Gradual onset
Rapid changes of the illness	Illness that evolves slowly
Heat	Cold
Restlessness, insomnia	Drowsiness, slowed attention
Throws off the covers	Wants to be covered up
Stretches out in bed	Curls up in bed
Warm body and limbs	Cold body and limbs
Red face	Pale face
Prefers cold drinks	Prefers hot drinks
Strong voice, talks a lot	Weak voice, prefers not to talk
Deep, strong breathing	Weak, superficial breathing,
Thirst	Absence of thirst
Scanty, dark urine	Abundant, pale urine
Constipation	Loose stools
Red tongue with yellow coating	Pale tongue

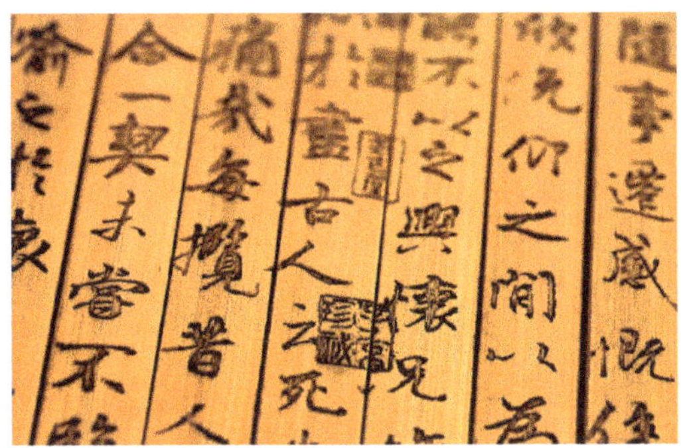

THE 6 ENERGY LEVELS

Qi is divided into three levels/aspects: **Tai** (greater, adult, maturity, maximum), **Shao** (lesser, youth, middle), **Jue** (terminal, senior, wisdom, minimum).
These energies flow through the body along the principle meridians that take their name from the energy level.

TAI YIN

The most superficial Yin that connects to Yang.
The mother, receptivity; Earth that opens herself to receive the energy from Heaven.
Quality: reflection, deliberation, depth, receptiveness, ability to open up to others, etc.
Imbalance: heaviness, communication difficulties, shutting out etc.

Lung (Shou Tai Yin) - Spleen (Zu Tae Yin)

SHAO YIN

A deeper form of Yin. The most intimate.
The source of life. The origin of Water (Yin) and Fire (Yang).
Quality: the ability to seduce, vitality, open heart, motivation, inner strength, etc.
Imbalance: introversion, shutting out, depression, etc.

Heart (Shou Shao Yin) – Kidney (Zu Shao Yin)

JUE YIN

Connects the Tai and the Shao Yin. The end of the Yin that leaves space for the Yang.
Completion, end.
Quality: openness to others, communication, etc.
Imbalance: submission, inability to battle on, giving up easily, etc.

Pericardium (Shou Jue Yin) - Liver (Zu Jue Yin)

TAI YANG

The great Yang. The most Yang of Yang. The most superficial.
The father, who sustains, makes rules and gives direction.
It represents an opening to the outside and it is the first defensive energy the body has against external attacks.
Quality: framework, organizational skills, structure, completeness, etc.
Imbalances: sense of confusion, blockage, rigidity, etc.

Small Intestine (Shou Tai Yang) - Bladder (Zu Tai Yang)

SHAO YANG

Connects the most superficial level of energy (Tai Yang) with the deepest level of energy (Yang Ming) and the various parts of the body.
It also regulates the flow of Yang energy throughout the whole body.
Quality: dynamism, vitality, communication skills, sense of justice, kindness, etc.
Imbalances: restlessness, a feeling of disorientation, contradiction, etc.

Triple Burner (Shou Shao Yang) - Gall Bladder (Zu Shao Yang)

YANG MING

Connects to the most superficial Yin.
It represents the deepest form of Yang that protects, preserves, purifies and transforms Qi.
Quality: introspection, reflection, integration, etc.
Imbalances: excessive defence, difficulties with learning and assimilation, etc.

Large Intestine (Shou Yang Ming) - Stomach (Zu Yang Ming)

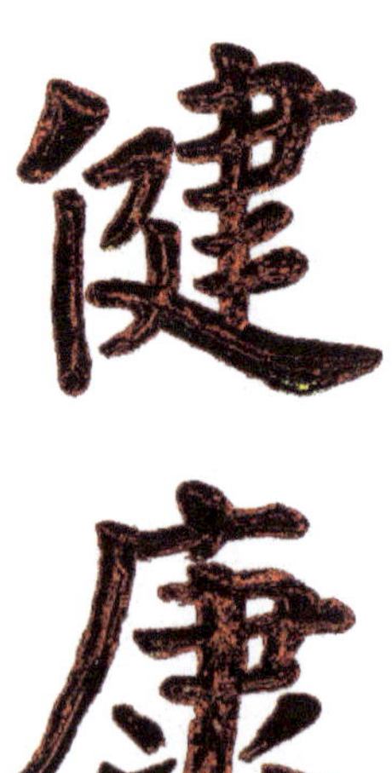

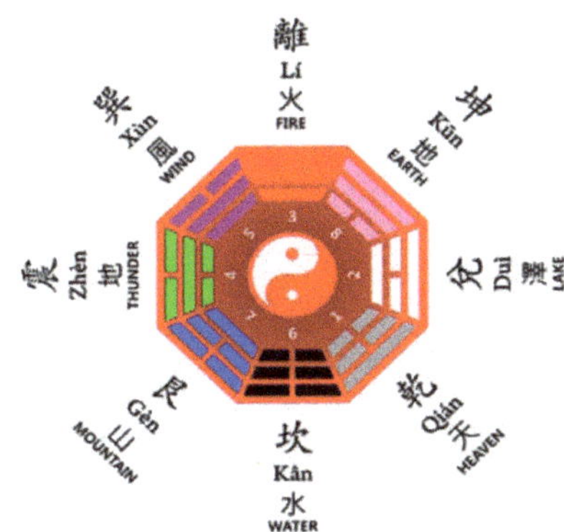

YIN	YANG
TAI YIN	**TAI YANG** (associated with Wei Qi)
LU - SP (Shou and Zu Tai Yin)	**SI – BL** (Shou and Zu Tai Yang)
Damp	**Cold**
SHAO YIN	**SHAO YANG**
HT - KD (Shou and Zu Shao Yin)	**TB – GB** (Shou and Zu Shao Yang)
Heat	**Fire**
JUE YIN	**YANG MING**
PC - LV (Shou and Zu Jue Yin)	**LI - ST** (Shou and Zu Yang Ming)
Wind	**Dryness**

Shou = arm

Zu = leg

<u>WATER</u>

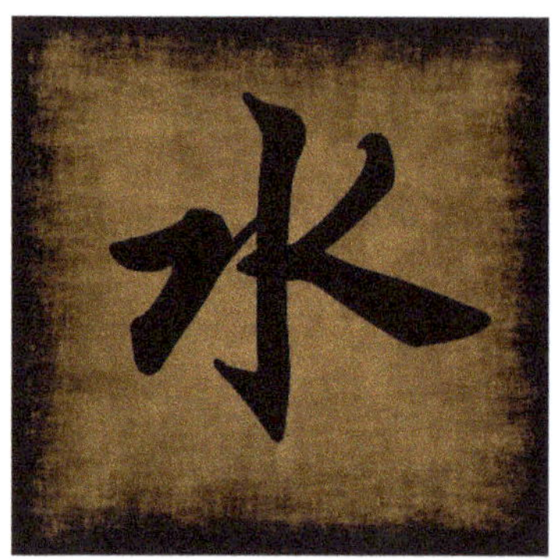

MOVEMENT:	DOWNWARDS
YIN-YANG:	VERY YIN/MAXIMUM YIN
DIRECTION:	NORTH
SEASON:	WINTER
PATHOGENIC FACTOR:	COLD
EVOLUTION:	ACCUMULATION – STORAGE
ORGAN:	KIDNEY
VISCERA:	BLADDER
COLOUR:	BLUE – BLACK
EMOTION:	FEAR
SPIRITUAL RESOURCE:	WILL POWER
SOUND:	GROAN, MOAN
CHARACTERISTIC:	TO TREMBLE
SENSE:	HEARING
SENSE ORGAN:	EARS
TISSUES:	BONES AND BONE MARROW
BODY FLUIDS:	SALIVA, SPIT, URINE
ORIFICES:	GENITALS, URETHRA, ANUS
EXTERNAL PHYSICAL MANIFESTATION:	HAIR
TASTE:	SALTY
ODOUR:	PUTRID
PLANET:	MERCURY
ANIMALS:	TURTLE
NUMBERS:	1-6

Water is the source of life.
It flows, hydrates and purifies.
Its nature is to flow downwards and fill every space it encounters.
It transports substances, nourishment.
It may be clear or cloudy, gentle and powerful, it can flow or stagnate.
The human body is mainly made up of water and this element governs the more internal parts of the body (spinal cord, brain, bones and bone marrow).
If there is an imbalance in the Water element, it can cause an imbalance in every aspect of the Body-Mind-Spirit.

IMBALANCES:

- Weakness in the joints.
- Dryness and thirst.
- Frequency or infrequency of urination.
- Excess or deficiency of perspiration.
- Kidney disease.
- Reduced metabolism.
- High or low blood pressure.
- Hypertension, phobias, nervousness.
- Sexual weakness, infertility.
- Swelling in the joints.
- Rheumatism, arthritis.
- Tooth decay.
- Depression, blocked emotions and thoughts, apathy.
- Fear, trepidation, coldness, shyness.
- Lack of will power,
- Lack of determination.
- Inability to face risk.
- Vertigo, dizziness, loss of balance.
- Noises, like the sound of a waterfall.
- Bone and bone marrow problems.
- Balding.

POSITIVE MENTAL STATES:

- Wisdom
- Intelligence.
- Reflectiveness
- Willpower, ambition.
- Determination.

COLOUR: BLUE / BLACK
Colours reminiscent of night and darkness.
In the case of a Water imbalance, you may notice that the face will have a bluish / blackish
complexion, especially around the eyes (associated with kidney dysfunction).
Often blue and black are the colours the person most prefers.

SEASON: WINTER
The maximum of Yin.
During this season it is important that the person conserves their energy as a seed does in
nature; resting and preserving the essence of life, preparing for the rebirth of spring.
It is a moment of silence.
If there is a Water imbalance, symptoms may become worse during the winter and this
season may prove to be unbearable.

CLIMATE: COLD
Excess cold causes many diseases and disorders related to Kidney and Bladder.
During the winter, it is important to conserve heat in the area of the kidneys so that the
Yang and the Fire of the Ancestral Qi preserved within can carry out their function of
warming the body.

TASTE: SALTY
Too much salt in the system causes fluid retention and therefore not recommended for
those suffering from high blood pressure.
Eating too much salty food is bad for the blood.
Salts control the hydro-saline balance through the functions of the kidneys.

ODOUR: ROTTEN
The smell of stagnant water.

EMOTION: FEAR
"Extreme fear can damage the Kidneys, but it can be counteracted by contemplation" (Nei
Ching).
Any type of phobia, obsessive or neurotic fear, but also feelings of fear, foreboding, anxiety.
Fear as in an inability to let go of anxieties, to fall into the depths of despair.
It is also the fear linked to the survival instinct, which in response to an emergency
situation causes a release of Kidney Ancestral Qi (adrenaline).

VOCAL QUALITY: MOANING GROANING
The voice of the person is constantly complaining.

CHARACTERISTIC: TREMBLING
Shaking as a release of withheld tension or as a natural response to tension caused by a
severe fright.

ORIFICE: GENITAL, URETHRA, ANUS
Much of the sexual function depends on a balance of the Water element.
Healthy reproduction, the functioning of the testes and ovaries, the flow of energy
necessary to perform the sexual act, as well as the lubrication, not only sperm but also of
the ova, depends on a good balance in the Water element.
The environment essential for the development of the embryo is water.
Often sexual problems can be directly attributed to a Water imbalance (impotence, sterility,
frigidity).
There are specific points on the Bladder and Kidney meridians that are directly related to
the sexual function and reproduction (D. M. Connelly 'Traditional Acupuncture').

SENSE ORGANS: EARS
Hearing, one of the first senses to develop in the foetus.
There are many acupuncture points on the ears that correspond to the embryonic
development of organs.
A Water imbalance can cause disorders such as labyrinthitis, vertigo, loss of balance, etc.

TISSUES: BONES AND BONE MARROW
All bones, including teeth (called 'the bones of the mouth'), draw nourishment from the
energy of Kidney and Bladder.
The cells that carry nourishment, strength and renewal to the all parts of the body are
regenerated in the bone marrow.
Even the spinal cord and brain (called the 'Sea of Marrow') are governed by the element
Water (Kidney).
Bone marrow nourishes the body through the blood, while the brain fuels thought
processes, attention, awareness, memory, mental clarity.
'The Kidney stores the Qi of the bones and the marrow' (Huangdi Neijing).
All bone problems are related to an imbalance of the Water element (tooth decay,
osteoporosis, etc.).

EXTERNAL PHYSICAL MANIFESTATION: HAIR
Strong, healthy hair reflects good Jing.
All problems related to the hair (hair loss, weakness, split ends, etc.) may be due to a Water
imbalance.

SPIRITUAL MANIFESTATION: WILL POWER
The Kidney stores Jing, the life force, impetus.
Water imbalance can manifest itself in a lack of willpower, lack of motivation, apathy,
fatigue, and difficulty in coping with even the simplest tasks.

<u>WOOD</u>

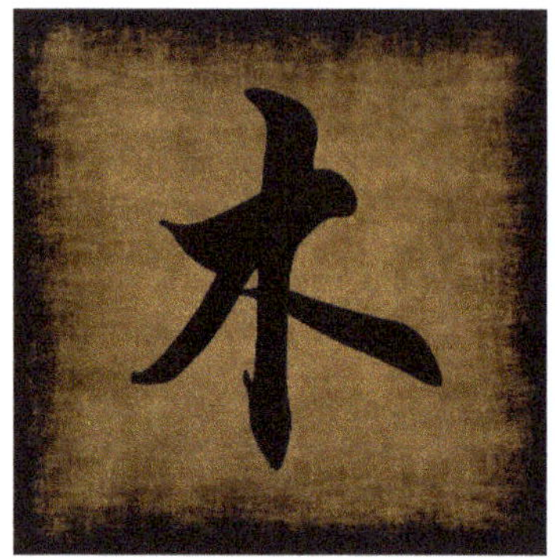

MOVEMENT: EXPANSION /IN ALL DIRECTIONS
YIN-YANG: YANG MINOR
DIRECTION: EAST
SEASON: SPRING
PATHOGENIC FACTOR: WIND
EVOLUTION: BIRTH
ORGAN: LIVER
VISCERA: GALL BLADDER
COLOUR: GREEN
EMOTION: ANGER / RAGE
SPIRITUAL RESOURCE: SPIRITUALITY
SOUND: SHOUTING
CHARACTERISTIC: TO CONTROL
SENSE: SIGHT
SENSE ORGAN: EYES
TISSUE: MUSCLES AND JOINTS
BODY FLUID: TEARS
ORIFICE: EYES
EXTERNAL PHYSICAL MANIFESTATION: NAILS
TASTE: SOUR / ACID
ODOUR: RANCID
PLANET: JUPITER
ANIMALS: FISH
NUMBERS: 3-8

Rebirth of nature after winter.
Transition from Yin to Yang, from darkness to light, from cold to heat.
The primary force that organizes life and growth.
Expansion towards the outside and in all directions.
Wood element is compared to the energy that allows the seed (guarded by the earth during the winter), to germinate and develop into a tree, becoming rooted, spreading up and out, remaining flexible, strong and resistant.
It is associated with any starting point, the birth of anything, our ability to adapt (the beginning of a relationship, a project, a job, the day, etc.).
The menstrual cycle is associated with the Wood element for its aspect of 'giving life' to the woman, the start of her reproductive life.

IMBALANCES:

- Lack of grounding that leads to falling easily, loss of balance.
- Rigidity (paralysis, arthritis, cramps, weakness of the limbs, etc.).
- Lack of flexibility of the spine.
- Visual disturbances.
- Irritability, anger, repression of emotions.
- Indecision, inability to organize, to plan, make decisions.
- Difficulty in falling asleep before 3am.

POSITIVE MENTAL STATES:

- Generosity, kindness, friendliness.
- Romantic love.
- Ability to decide, plan and organize.
- Capacity to coordinate, cooperate and control.
- Creativity.
- Patience.
- Adaptability, flexibility.

COLOUR: GREEN
Colour of Spring, nature that awakens and revives.
Green is the colour of bile.

SEASON: SPRING
Spring is the best time to detoxify the body.

CLIMATE: WIND
"The Wind is the cause of a hundred diseases" (Nei Ching).
Wind is such a dynamic and penetrating climatic influence that, if incurred in excess, it can lead to acute inflammation in the body.
Depressive illnesses can also worsen due to an excess of Wind.
TCM often mentions Internal Wind; a condition caused by an imbalance of the Liver and Gall Bladder, characterized by symptoms that move in a confused way, changing suddenly and appearing and disappearing for no apparent reason.

DIRECTION: EAST
"Beginning and creation come from the East" (Nei Ching).

TASTE: SOUR / ACID
The sour/acid taste has an astringent effect and an excess hardens the flesh.

ODOUR: RANCID
A strong smell, disgusting, fetid, as urine or acid sweat.

EMOTION: ANGER / RAGE
A Wood imbalance can manifest itself with outbursts of anger, excessive anger or a complete inability to externalise feelings.
Repressed anger leads to frustration and inner conflict and often turns into depression.
Even repressed creativity can create anger, imbalance and depression.
An excess of anger affects Liver and Gall Bladder, although by expressing anger everything passes through the nervous system and as a result all organs are compromised.

SOUND: SHOUT
An aggressive, penetrating tone of voice, to attract attention, like a cry for help, is without doubt indicative of a Wood imbalance.

CHARACTERISTIC: CAPACITY TO CONTROL
Coordination, planning, decision-making skills, organizational, etc.

ORIFICE: EYES
"When the Liver receives blood, this strengthens sight" (Nei Ching).

SENSE ORGAN: EYES
"The eye must shine with perception" (Nei Ching).
A Wood imbalance can cause problems to the eyes and sight.
It can even manifest itself as a distorted view of life, of a situation or a period of time,
which can be the cause of inappropriate behaviour or of poor decision making.

BODY TISSUE: Muscles, ligaments and tendons
"The Liver houses the life force of muscles and tissues (tendons and ligaments)" (Nei Ching).
A Wood imbalance can lead to extreme fatigue that affects the muscles and tendons, i.e the connective tissue that gives elasticity and strength to the muscles and attaches them firmly to the bones.
Therefore, all muscle and tendon disorders (sprains, injuries, etc.) are attributed to the condition of the energy of the Wood element.

EXTERNAL PHYSICAL MANIFESTATION: NAILS
"The condition of the nails demonstrates when the Liver is in a splendid and flourishing condition" (Nei Ching).
When there is a Liver Blood deficiency, the nails are brittle. Redness, stains, flaking, cracks, undulations on nails, etc. are manifestations of the condition of Liver.

SPIRITUAL MANIFESTATION: SPIRITUALITY
In TCM the ethereal soul or spirit (Hun) resides in the Liver, as do the emotions.
Hun is understood as 'the soul we put into what we do'.

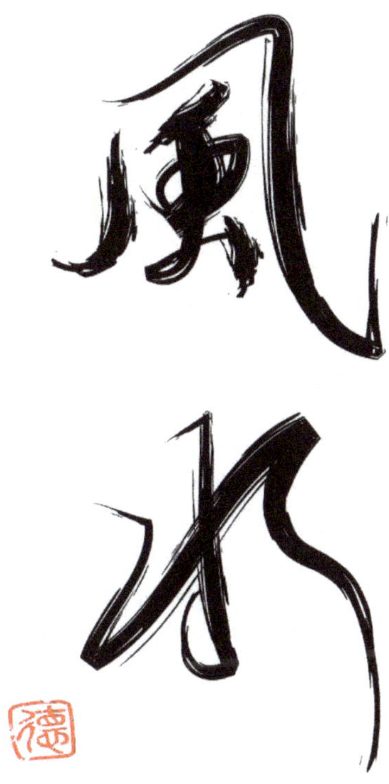

FIRE

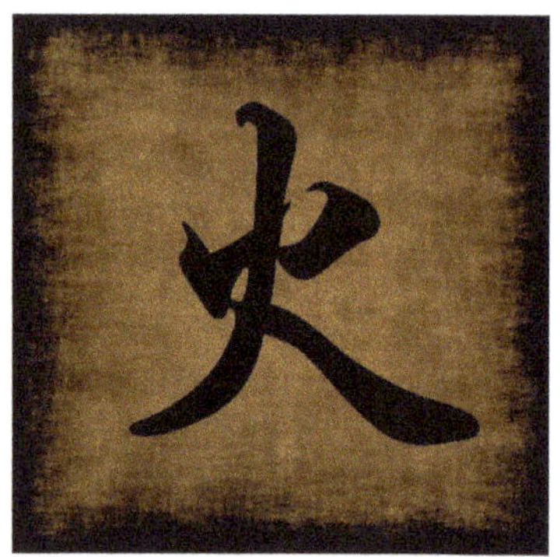

MOVEMENT:	UPWARDS
YIN-YANG:	MAXIMUM YANG
DIRECTION:	SOUTH
SEASON:	SUMMER
PATHOGENIC FACTOR:	HEAT
EVOLUTION:	GROWTH, SUMMIT
ORGANS:	HEART – PERICARDIUM
VISCERA:	SMALL INTESTINE - TRIPLE HEATER
COLOUR:	RED
EMOTION:	JOY
SPIRITUAL RESOURCE:	MEDITATION, WISDOM, STRENGTH
SOUND:	LAUGHTER
CHARACTERISTICS:	INTERPRETATION, ABSORPTION, CIRCULATION, PROTECTION
SENSE ORGAN:	TONGUE
TISSUES:	BLOOD VESSELS
BODY FLUID:	SWEAT
ORIFICE:	EARS
EXTERNAL PHYSICAL MANIFESTATION:	COMPLEXION
TASTE:	BITTER
ODOUR:	SCORCHED
PLANET:	MARS
ANIMALS:	BIRDS
NUMBERS:	2-7

Fire burns and rises; it is heat, light, vitality, but also destruction.
It is a dynamic and transforming force.
It is the most Yang of all the elements.
It is the only element that has two pairs of meridians - (Heart / Small Intestine and Pericardium / Triple Burner).
Fire, more than any other element, governs social interaction.

IMBALANCES

- Fevers.
- Lack of emotional warmth.
- Sexual frigidity (Fire that has gone out).
- Poor blood circulation (cold extremities, varicose veins, haemorrhoids, hot flushes, etc.).
- Heartburn and digestive problems.
- Hyperactivity, confusion, impulsiveness, recklessness.
- Inability to finish what you started.
- Loss of sensation in a limb.
- General sense of malaise in which you feel you just can't get anything done.

POSITIVE MENTAL STATES

- Courtesy.
- Courage.
- Fervour.
- Joy.
- Love.
- Awareness.

COLOUR: RED

"When their colour is red like blood, they are without life" (Nei Ching).
When there is a Fire imbalance the face will appear red or completely absent of any red hue (ashen).
Even the tendency to blush easily is linked to an imbalance in this element (the heart responds too readily to emotional stimuli).

SEASON: SUMMER

The maximum Yang.
The period of vigorous growth, the hottest season of the year; the culmination of the annual growth of nature.

This whole process of completion and maturation includes the thought process, experience, the body and emotions.

CLIMATE: HEAT
Excessive heat can alter the balance in the Fire element.

DIRECTION: SOUTH
"Nutrition and growth come from the South" (Nei Ching).

TASTE: BITTER
"The heart desires the bitter taste" (Nei Ching).
Bitter tasting substances can clear the heart.
The bitter taste has a strengthening effect.
Many vegetables, coffee, dark chocolate, and anything toasted are bitter, as well as the flavour of herbs.
A Fire imbalance can bring about a bitter taste in the mouth.

ODOUR: SCORCHED
This burnt smell is quite understandable given that it is the odour associated with the Fire element.

EXCITEMENT: JOY
Expression of harmony of the Shen.
An excess or the total lack of joy are equally harmful.
An imbalance of this emotion easily affects the social life of the person.

SOUND: LAUGHTER
"An excess of Shen is a laugh that is not quenched" (Nei Ching).
It may be a subtle laugh, evasive, just a hint of a laugh, which manifests itself continuously, even in a sad conversation, like a need to ease the embarrassment.
It can also be an exaggerated laughter or inappropriate laughter.
Even the complete absence of laughter is associated with a Fire imbalance.

SPIRITUAL CHARACTERISTIC: CAPACITY TO FEEL SADNESS AND PAIN
Learn to accept, recognize and embrace the experiences in life that bring sadness and pain.

ORIFICE: EARS
The Fire meridians (TB and SI) pass near the ears.

SENSE ORGAN: TONGUE
"The Heart rules the tongue" (Nei Ching).

From looking at the tongue we can obtain information about the heart and blood circulation.

The tongue, as a speech organ, through which the heart can express itself.
A Fire imbalance can cause problems relating to speech (stuttering, muteness, logorrhoea, etc.).
Ulcers on the tongue indicate a pathogenic Heat in the Heart.

TISSUES: BLOOD VESSELS
Problems related to circulation (hardening of the arteries, varicose veins, cold extremities, thrombosis, etc.) are all symptoms of Fire imbalance.

BODY FLUID: SWEAT
Sweat is considered healthy, because through it the body has a means to expel toxins and cleanse itself.

EXTERNAL PHYSICAL MANIFESTATION: COMPLEXION
The Fire element reflects in the face (complexion, quality, etc.)

VITAL CHARACTERISTIC: THE SHEN
Shen resides in the Heart.

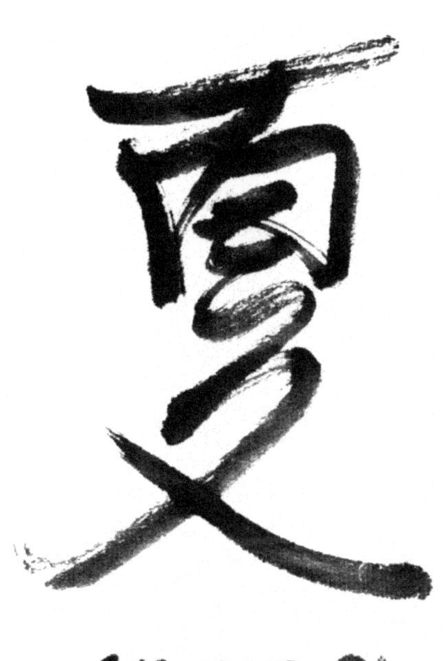

EARTH

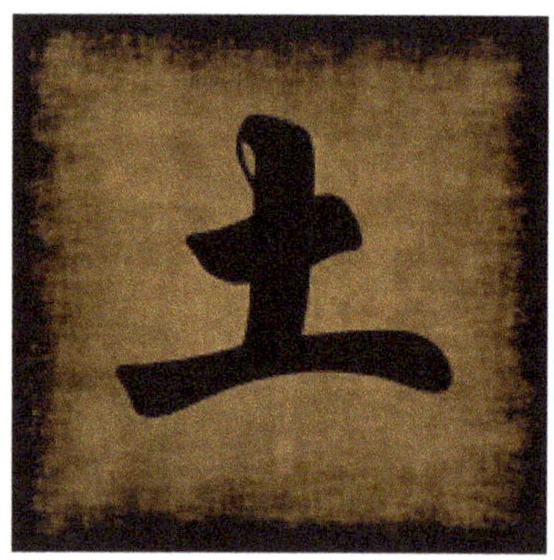

MOVEMENT:	NEUTRALITY – STABILITY
YIN-YANG:	CENTRE
DIRECTION:	CENTRE
SEASON:	LATE SUMMER
PATHOGENIC FACTOR:	DAMPNESS
EVOLUTION:	TRANSFORMATION
ORGANS:	SPLEEN / PANCREAS
VISCERA:	STOMACH
COLOUR:	YELLOW
EMOTION:	COMPASSION - SYMPATHY - EMPATHY – CONCERN
CAPACITY:	IDEAS AND OPINIONS
SOUND:	SING
CHARACTERISTIC:	BELCHING
SENSE:	TASTE
SENSE ORGAN:	MOUTH
TISSUES:	MUSCLES
BODY FLUID:	SALIVA
ORIFICES:	MOUTH
TASTE:	SWEET
ODOUR:	FRAGRANT
PLANET:	SATURN
ANIMALS:	HUMAN BEINGS
NUMBERS:	5-10

The Earth receives the seed and nourishes it; it is the womb that welcomes life.
The Mother.
The qualities that characterize it are: stability, strength, support, nurturing, reliability, fullness, centred, fertility, receptivity, balance, acceptance.
The Earth is the centre from which all elements come and where they are nourished.
Its fundamental function is to receive food and transform it into energy.
A good connection with the Earth helps us to deal with changes while remaining centred and receptive.

Stomach and Spleen, the two Earth meridians, have a very close relationship.

IMBALANCES:

- Give and take: inability to find the right balance between these two aspects.
- Loss of natural rhythms: menstruation, hormonal, sleep, breath, seasons, thought processes harmony and body coordination.
- Ulcers, indigestion, obesity, vomiting, abdominal bloating, hyperacidity, spastic pains.
- Anorexia and bulimia.
- Dry lips, bleeding gums.
- Amenorrhea, dysmenorrhea.
- Nervousness, fickleness, instability, loss of balance, insecurity.
- Depends on the presence of others.
- Selfishness.
- Weight problems (poor distribution of Earth energy).
- Infertility.
- Mid-morning hunger pangs.
- Diarrhoea and constipation.

POSITIVE MENTAL STATES:

- Empathy.
- Desire to take care of.
- Sympathy.

COLOUR: YELLOW
The colour of ripe cereal.
In diagnosis, you check for any yellow colouring around the mouth.

SEASON: LATE SUMMER
In fact, the Earth does not correspond to one season in particular, but rather to a short period at the end of each season, when energy returns to the Centre to be regenerated. These moments of transition between one season and the other are often accompanied by adverse climatic changes that lead to an increase in dampness which is a characteristic associated with Earth.
Particular sensitivity to seasonal changes indicates an imbalance in the Earth element.

CLIMATE: DAMP
Excess Dampness can cause an imbalance in the energy of the Earth element, as can the total absence of Dampness (dryness).

DIRECTION: CENTRE
"Everything that is created by the Universe meets in the Centre and is absorbed by the Earth" (Nei Ching).
The Centre symbolizes stability, balance, neutrality.

TASTE: SWEET
The taste of cereals, root vegetables, food that is in contact with the earth.

ODOUR: SWEET – FRAGRANT
A sweet smell, almost nauseating.

EMOTION: SYMPATHY, COMPASSION, CONCERN, EMPATHY
The ability to be compassionate, to find a balance between giving and receiving.
Knowing how to reflect and have self-discipline, to have self-confidence and be able to trust in others.

SOUND: SINGING
A singsong tone, melodious chirping.
The person speaks in a 'singing' fashion.

CHARACTERISTIC: BELCHING
Belching and hiccupping.
Excessive belching and hiccupping frequently indicates an imbalance in the Earth element.

SENSE ORGAN: MOUTH
Food and air both enter the body via the mouth.
The lips provide information about the state of Stomach and Spleen energy (texture, elasticity, firmness, moisture, etc.).
Various oral addictions (eating, smoking, alcohol, etc.) can indicate an Earth imbalance.

BODY FLUID: SALIVA
Lack or excess of saliva.
Problems swallowing.

TISSUE: FLESH
"The life force of the flesh lives in the Spleen" (Nei Ching).
"When the Spleen is healthy it can generate all living things".
The condition of the flesh (texture, tone, temperature, etc.) indicates whether a person is lacking in nourishment.

CAPACITY: IDEAS AND OPINIONS
Capacity for introspection.
To have an inspiration, opinions, and ideas and be able to bring them to fruition.

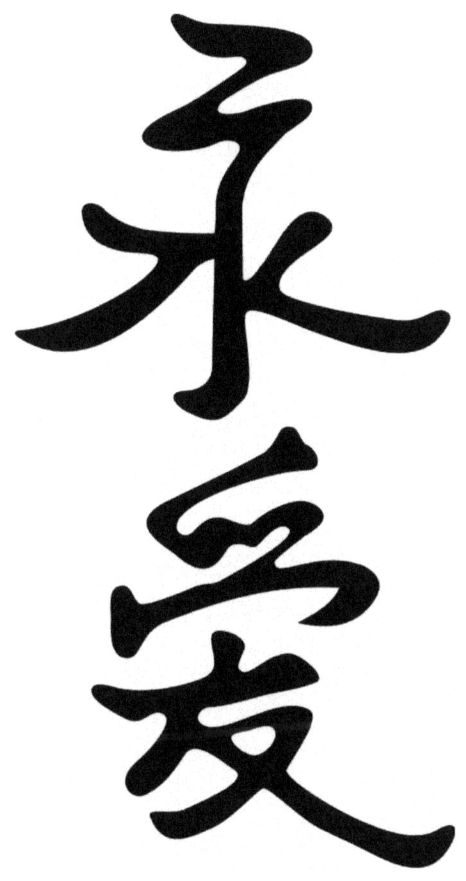

<u>METAL</u>

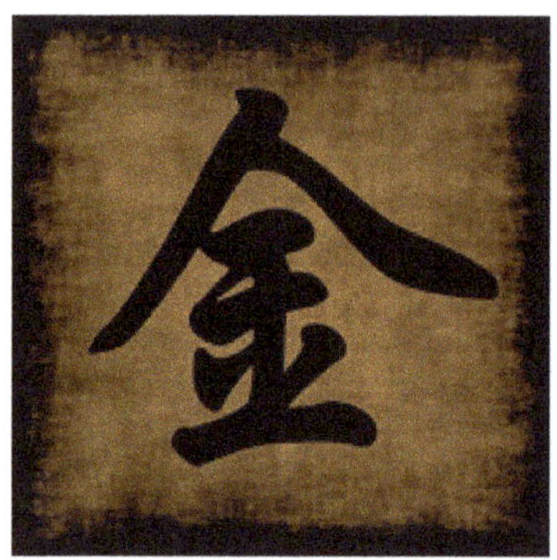

MOVEMENT:	TOWARDS THE INTERIOR
YIN-YANG:	YIN MINOR
DIRECTION:	WEST
SEASON:	AUTUMN
PATHOGENIC FACTOR:	DRYNESS
EVOLUTION:	HARVEST
ORGANS:	LUNGS
VISCERA:	LARGE INTESTINE
COLOUR:	WHITE
EMOTION:	SADNESS
SOUND:	CRYING
CHARACTERISTIC:	COUGHING
SENSE:	SMELL
SENSORY ORGAN:	NOSE
TISSUES:	SKIN AND HAIR
BODY FLUID:	MUCOUS
EXTERNAL MANIFESTATION:	SKIN AND HAIR
TASTE:	SPICY
ODOUR:	PUNGENT – ROTTEN
PLANET:	VENUS
ANIMALS:	MAMMALS
NUMBERS:	4-9

The exact translation of the Chinese character for Metal is 'gold', so, a precious metal, durable, unaffected by the elements, pliant.

Metal as in minerals that provide the earth with substances, richness, structure, preciousness.

Metal is also a conductor of electricity, so it symbolizes communication, exchange, the ability to socialise.

One of the qualities of Metal is its ability to take any shape or form.

It can melt and harden again, change its state and return to its previous state; for this reason it is associated with the ability to develop ways of thinking that are steadfast but flexible and with the ability to create harmonious exchanges with the outside world.

IMBALANCES:

- Rheumatic pains.
- Degeneration or a stiffness of the spine.
- Tremors.
- Spasms of the throat, oesophagus.
- Some types of paralysis.
- Debilitating diseases.
- Lack of emotional strength.
- Incoherence in speech.
- Rashes, psoriasis, acne.
- Allergies, asthma.
- Colitis (inflammation of the intestinal mucous membrane).
- Spastic colon.
- Intestinal problems.
- Autism.
- Depression.
- Insecurity.
- Isolation.
- Sense of emptiness and lack of self-esteem.
- Perfectionism.

POSITIVE MENTAL STATES:

- Feel connected to the outside world.
- Self-esteem.
- Ability to change, be flexible.
- Communication.
- Ability to establish relationships.

COLOUR: WHITE
Pale face (Lung Qi deficiency).
In the East it is used as the colour of mourning.

SEASON: AUTUMN
Transition from Yin to Yang, from light to dark, from hot to cold.
The gathering of energy, time for reflection, and internalization.

CLIMATE: DRYNESS
Anyone who has an excessive love or hate of the dry climate, anyone who have excessively
dry skin may have a Metal imbalance.
Excessive dryness is harmful to the lungs.

DIRECTION: WEST
"Precious metals and jade come from the regions of the West" (Nei Ching).

TASTE: SPICY
"An excess of spicy food makes muscles knotted and makes nails dry and spoil. When you
have a disease in the respiratory tract you should not eat too much spicy food" (Nei Ching).
The spicy flavour activates perspiration, opens pores and promotes the circulation of fluid
secretions and the distribution of Qi.

ODOUR: ROTTEN
A smell of something rotting.

EMOTION: SADNESS
A good Metal energy makes it possible to welcome even sadness and pain, to overcome
them and not remain trapped by them.
After a difficult and painful period a person may suffer from bowel problems and / or
difficulty breathing.
A person who is unable to express sadness and pain and, because these emotions are
considered unacceptable, represses them, may show a Metal imbalance.

SOUND: CRYING
A tearful voice, plaintive.
Crying easily or repression of crying indicates a Metal imbalance.

CHARACTERISTIC: COUGHING
Coughing manifests the need to expel something unwanted (both physically and
emotionally).

SENSE ORGAN: NOSE
The nose is clearly connected to the lungs because you breathe through it, but it is also connected to the Large Intestine because its meridian pathway has two points at the base of the nose (see LI 19 and LI 20).
Dysfunctions in the sense of smell relate to a Metal imbalance.

BODY FLUID: MUCOUS
All problems concerning mucous (runny or stuffy nose, dry nose, frequent sneezing, sinus congestion, etc.) relate to a Metal imbalance.

TISSUES: SKIN AND HAIR
The skin is considered a third lung, therefore linked to the exchange with the outside world, but also as a means to eliminate toxins.
Through the skin (touch) we can communicate or perceive feelings and emotions.
Acne reflects, not only the need to excrete waste products, but also a difficulty in dealing with relationships, with the exchange with the outside world.

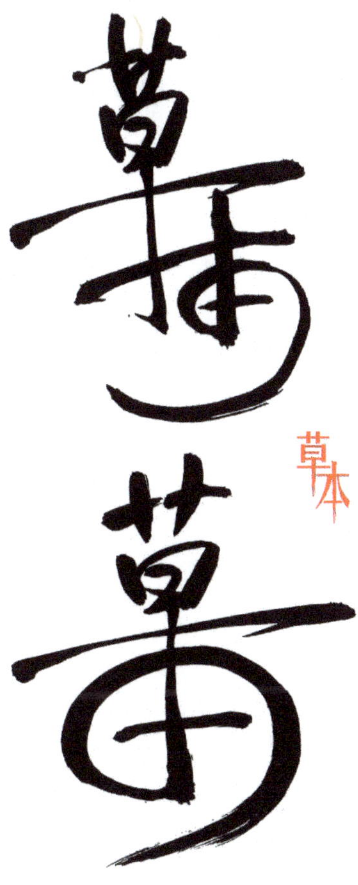

GENERATING SEQUENCE
(Sheng Cycle)

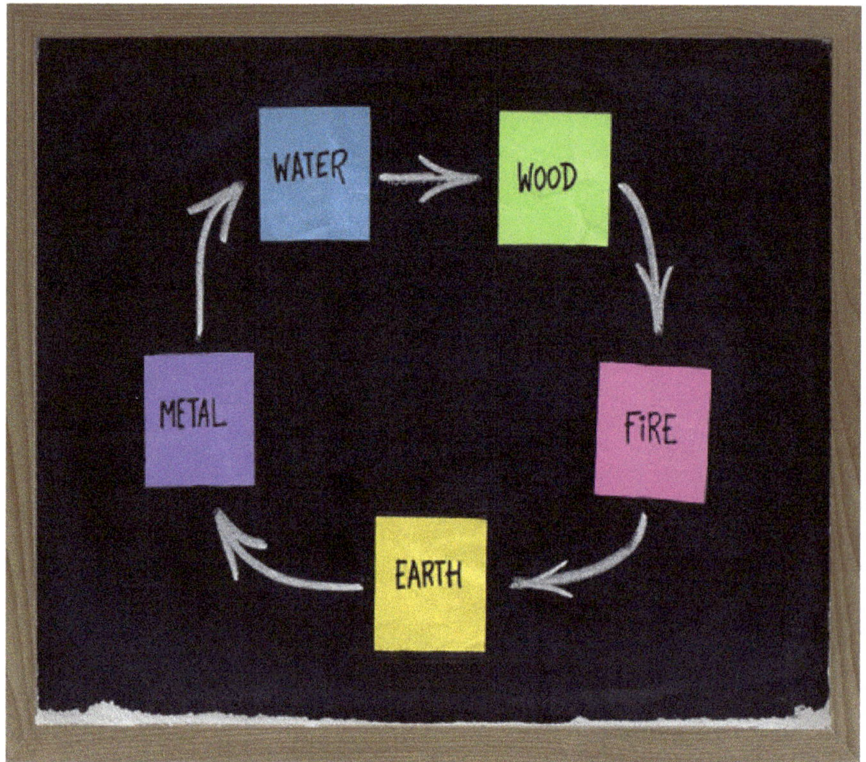

Each element generates another and, in turn, is generated by another.

Also called **'Mother-Child Cycle'.**

Wood creates Fire; Fire creates Earth (by reducing wood to ashes); Earth creates Metal (by becoming minerals, stones, etc.); Metal creates Water (supplying it with mineral salts) and Water creates Wood.
An imbalance in any one element is transmitted to the next.

Generating Sequence Imbalance:

When there is an organ deficiency due to a lack of nourishment from the Mother Element or vice versa:

1. The Mother is weak and cannot support the Child sufficiently.
2. The Child absorbs too much energy from the Mother.

WOOD FAILS TO NOURISH FIRE

If there is a Liver (which houses the Shen) Blood deficiency, it is unable to nourish the Heart.
If, on the other hand, there is a Gall Bladder deficiency, the Heart will be affected by this lack of courage and determination.

- insomnia (waking up early in the morning)
- palpitations
- lack of courage
- emotional weakness
- indecision
- shyness

FIRE AFFECTS WOOD

If there is a Heart-Blood deficiency, it can affect the ability of the Liver to accumulate it.

- scanty menstruation

FIRE FAILS TO NOURISH EARTH

The transformation functions of the Spleen may be compromised if the Heart is unable to pump the Blood (Empty Heart Fire). This condition can also affect the ability to concentrate.

- feeling cold and weakness in the limbs
- loose stools, diarrhoea
- asthenia

EARTH AFFECTS FIRE

If the Spleen does not produce enough Blood then the Heart suffers.

- insomnia

- palpitations

- poor memory

- slight depression

EARTH FAILS TO NOURISH METAL

Lungs need Spleen Qi to form Zong Qi.
If the functions of the Spleen are impaired, phlegm can build up in the lungs.

- asthenia

- phlegm in the Lungs

- difficulty breathing (dyspnoea)

- asthma

- cough

METAL AFFECTS EARTH

A Lung Qi deficiency can impair the Spleen Qi.

- lack of appetite

- loose stools

- tiredness

METAL FAILS TO CREATE WATER

The Lungs send Qi and fluid to the Kidneys, if this function is compromised it can lead to
Kidney dryness.

- difficulty breathing (dyspnoea)

- asthma

- cough

- loss of voice

WATER AFFECTS METAL

If there is a Kidney Qi deficiency, it cannot restrain Qi from rising upwards where it can congest the Lungs.

- difficulty breathing

WATER FAILS TO NOURISH WOOD

Liver Blood is nourished by Kidney Yin, but if there is a deficiency, a Yin and Liver Blood deficiency may result.

- headache

- dizziness

- tinnitus

- blurred vision

- irritability

WOODS AFFECTS WATER

If there is a Liver Blood deficiency over an extended period of time, it can cause a Kidney Jing deficiency.

- sexual weakness

- night sweats

- tinnitus

- dizziness

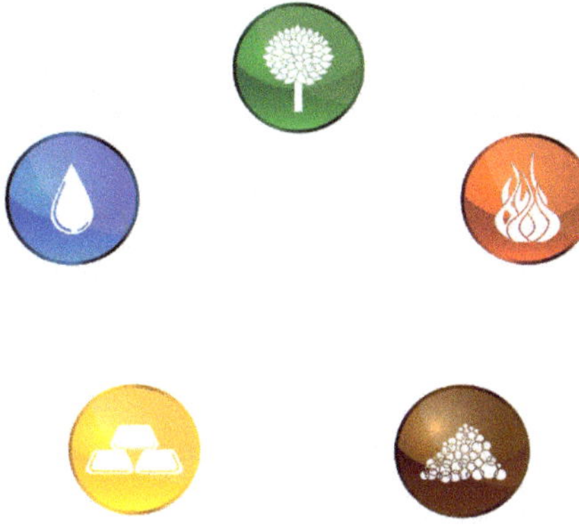

INHIBITING OR CONTROLLING SEQUENCE
(Ko Cycle)

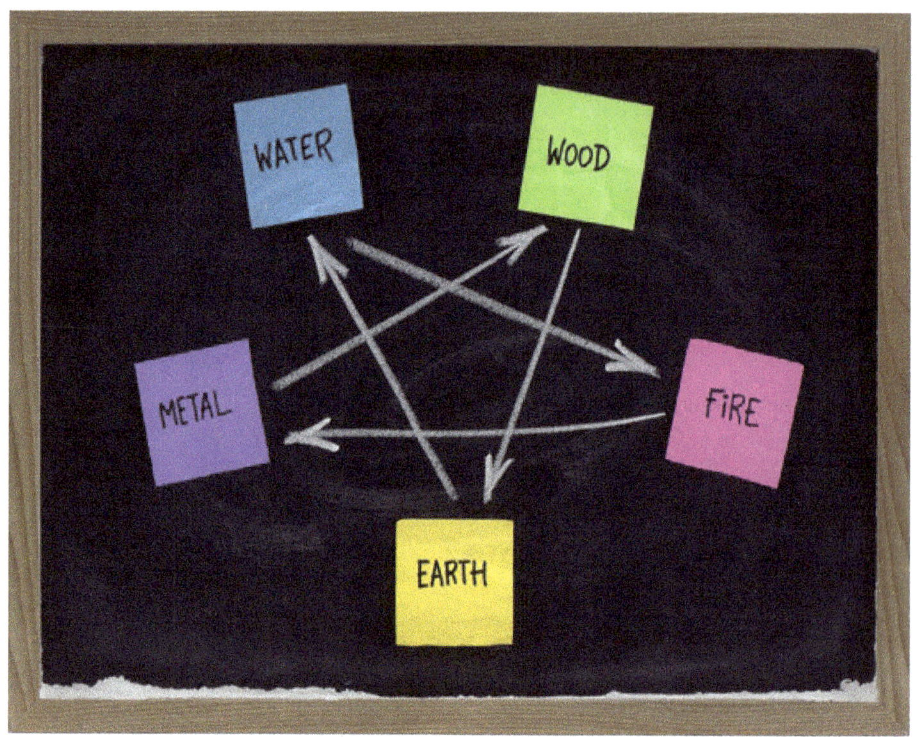

Each element controls the second element that follows it and is controlled by the second preceding it.

Also called **'Grandparent-Grandchild' relationship.**

Wood inhibits / controls the Earth (roots holding it/by covering it); Earth inhibits / controls Water (by absorbing, and forming riverbanks); Water inhibits / controls Fire (by putting it out); Fire inhibits / controls Metal (by melting it); Metal inhibits/controls Wood (by chopping it down).

OVERWHELMING SEQUENCE
(Cheng Cycle)

Each element is excessively controlled by the second that follows, damaging or draining it.

Overwhelming Cycle Imbalances:

WOOD OVERWHELMS EARTH

If Liver Qi stagnates, it can invade the Spleen and Stomach, preventing them from carrying out their food transformation functions and those relating to the movement of Qi (Stomach Qi to descend and Spleen Qi to ascend).

- diarrhoea

- epigastric pain

- bloated feeling

- irritability

- poor appetite

- nausea

EARTH OVERWHELMS WATER

In the case of an accumulation of Dampness, the Spleen blocks the Kidney functions of transformation and elimination of liquids.

- fluid retention, oedema

- difficulty in urination

WATER OVERWHELMS FIRE

This cannot happen, because Kidneys are never in a condition of Excess.
Kidney Yin deficiency can cause a condition of Empty Heart Heat.

<u>**FIRE OVERWHELMS METAL**</u>

Heart Fire can cause a Lung Yin Deficiency, drying out liquids.

- red face

- feeling of being hot

- cough with abundant yellow sputum

<u>**METAL OVERWHELMS WOOD**</u>

A Lung Deficiency can cause a stagnation of Liver Qi.

- pale face

- irritability

- bloated feeling

- asthenia

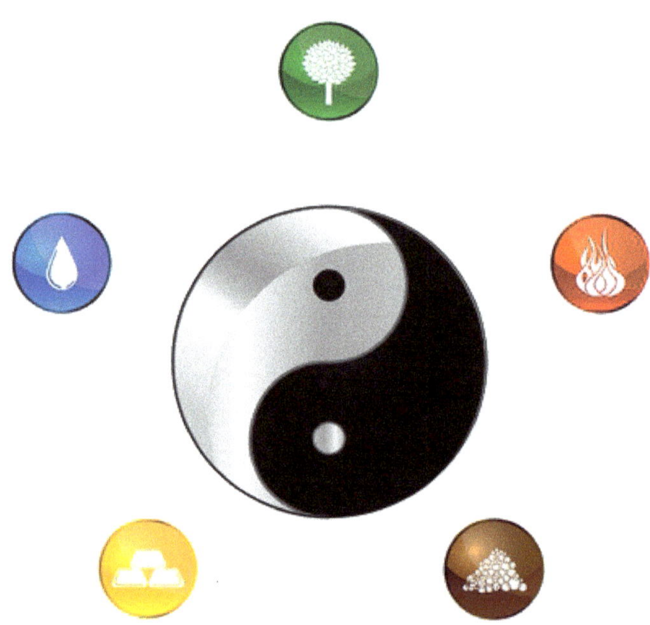

INSULTING SEQUENCE
(Wu Cycle)

It occurs in the opposite direction to that of the inhibiting sequence.

Insulting Sequence Imbalances:

WOOD INSULTS METAL

If Liver Qi stagnates in the upper part of the body, it can obstruct the chest and impair breathing.

- feeling of obstruction and swollen chest

- cough

- asthma

METAL INSULTS FIRE

If the lungs are obstructed by phlegm, the circulation of Heart Qi may be impeded.

- difficulty breathing

- palpitations

- insomnia

FIRE INSULTS WATER

Heart Fire descending can cause a Kidney Yin Deficiency.

- night sweats

- dry mouth at night

- insomnia

- back pain

- dizziness

<u>**WATER INSULTS EARTH**</u>

If the Kidneys do not effectively carry out their function of liquid transformation the Spleen can become blocked by Dampness.

- limb weakness

- asthenia

- oedema

- loose stools

<u>**EARTH INSULTS WOOD**</u>

If Spleen Dampness stagnates, this can hinder the flow of Liver Qi.

- pain and swelling in the abdomen

- jaundice

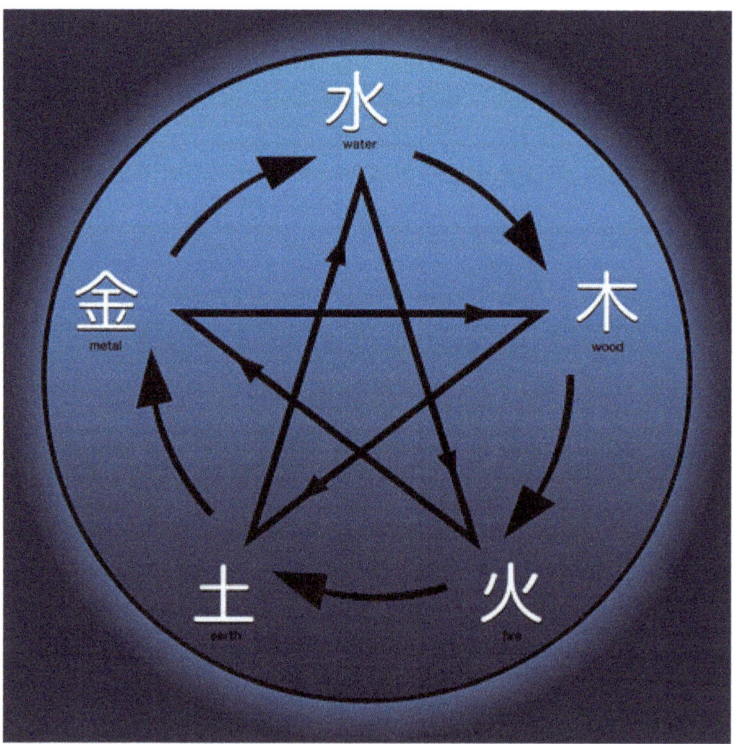

VITAL SUBSTANCES

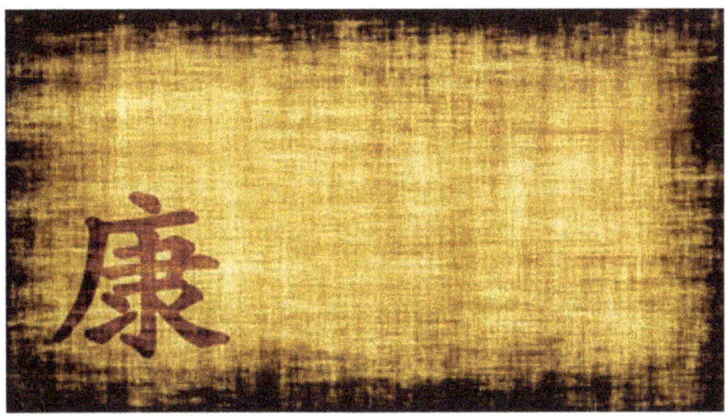

JING (Essence)

The force, power that is the material basis for all life and is consumed by our very existence.
Jing is the power of the union between Heaven and Earth; the root of Life.
A pure, precious, highly refined substance derived by distillation from a solid raw material
and which must be protected and preserved with care.

It is divided into:

Prenatal Jing (Pre-Heaven Essence)

Postnatal Jing (Post-Heaven Essence)

Kidney Jing

With our first breath the cosmic Qi (Tian Qi) is pushed down into the abdomen (Dan
Dien) by the Lungs where it joins with the Jing and establishes a Lung-Kidney connection.
At the same time, from the feet, Earth Qi rises and, it too, meets in the Dan Dien.
The powerful movement of these two forces creates a kind of vortex around the navel that
activates the Jing conserved by the Kidneys (Ming Men GV4, it is from this point that we
start to grow from the moment of conception) making it mobile and promoting its
circulation (Yuan Qi).

PRENATAL JING

Original energy, present from the moment of conception.
It is the condensation of cosmic energies that allows each individual to 'take shape'; the essence that arises from the union of the sexual energies of the parents and the cosmic union at the moment of conception.
It is the precious essence that nourishes the embryo and foetus during pregnancy and from birth onwards it must be conserved carefully for when it runs out, this coincides with the extinction of the individual's life, the 'losing shape'.
It is what determines the physical features of each person, their strength, vitality, and uniqueness.
It is the energy that we inherit from our parents (and ancestors).
The individual draws nourishment and sustenance from Prenatal Jing and slowly and inevitably it is gradually consumed.
Although it cannot be changed in quantity or quality, it can be conserved and consumed more slowly by striving for balance in our daily life and habits.
Every irregularity or excess in life activities can reduce it.

In summary:

- Governs growth, development and reproduction;

- Determines basic constitution, strength and vitality of the individual;

- Determines the activation of all organic metabolisms.

POSTNATAL JING

It is the energy that concerns all psycho-physical-energetic nutrition of the individual.
It develops after birth and is the essence that we obtain from outside the body through nutritional substances (food, water, air, interests, relationships, etc.).
If assimilation of the Postnatal Jing is good, the Prenatal Jing will be consumed at a slower rate and therefore be preserved longer.
However, there is a close relationship of mutual influence between the two, so, if an individual is born with a delicate and poorly functioning digestive system, the assimilation of Jing from food may be unsatisfactory or impaired.
Postnatal Jing also includes psychological and emotional nourishment, which we obtain from the external environment and from our thoughts.
It is quite clearly related to Spleen and Stomach, but also to Lung.

<u>**KIDNEY JING**</u>

It derives from both Prenatal and Postnatal Jing, from which it receives nourishment.
It is the hereditary energy that determines our constitution.
It is stored in the Kidneys, but being by nature fluid, it circulates throughout the body, particularly in the 8 Extraordinary Channels.
Kidney Jing determines conception, reproduction, pregnancy, growth, development and sexual maturity.
It is necessary for the transformation of the Kidney Yin to Kidney Qi through the heating action of the Kidney Yang.
It also has a Yang aspect that influences sexual activity and in particular the libido.
Jing produces Marrow, which generates bone marrow and "fills up" the spinal cord and brain.
Jing determines our constitutional strength and resistance to external pathogenic factors.

Kidney Jing Deficiency can cause:

- Problems related to growth, reproduction and development (slow growth in children, poor bone development, infertility, miscarriages, mental retardation in children, bone deterioration in adults, loss of teeth and hair, premature greying of the hair);

- Kidney Qi problems (poor sexual activity, impotence, weakness of the knees, nocturnal emission, tinnitus and deafness);

- Problems related to the Marrow (poor memory and concentration, dizziness, tinnitus and light-headedness);

- Constitutional problems (frequent colds, flu and other exogenous pathogenic influences, chronic and allergic rhinitis).

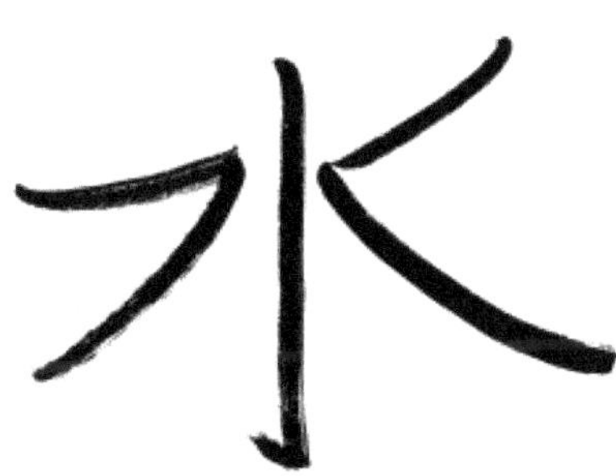

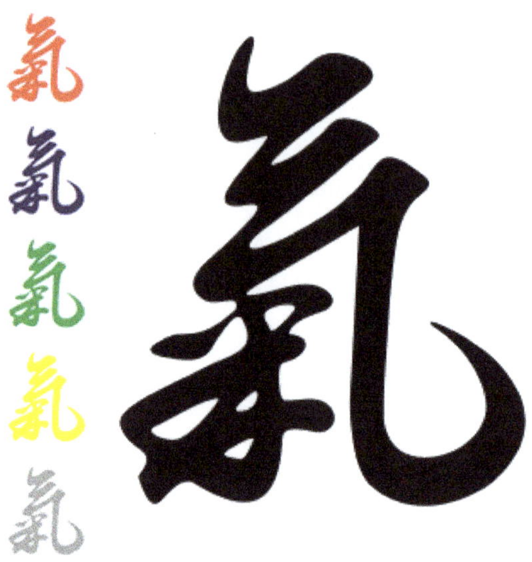

<u>QI (Energy)</u>

Qi can be rarefied and immaterial, or dense and material.
It has a changeable nature; it can manifest itself in many different ways and be different things at different times.
It is at the root of every phenomena in the universe and ensures continuity between the raw forms and materials and the non-material, fine, rarefied energies.
It is an energy that manifests itself simultaneously on both the physical and spiritual level.
It is in a constant state of flux and in various states of aggregation.
When it condenses, the energy transforms and accumulates in physical forms.
Qi changes its form depending on its location and the function it is carrying out.
It has two main aspects: it constitutes the refined essence produced by the internal organs to nourish the body and mind (Zong Qi, Yuan Qi, etc.) and also represents the functional activity of the internal organs (Liver Qi, Heart Qi, etc.).
The individual Qi represents activation, transformation and distribution of all that is derived from Jing and that returns to it.
Qi is the intermediate element between Jing and Shen (nourished by the Qi produced by the body to then return again to Jing and Shen).

It is divided into:

Yuan Qi	-	**Ancestral / Original Qi**
Gu Qi	-	**Food Qi**
Zong Qi	-	**Gathering Qi or Qi of the Chest**
Zhen Qi	-	**True Qi**
Ying Qi	-	**Nutritive Qi**
Wei Qi	-	**Protective Qi**

<u>YUAN QI (Ancestral/Original Qi)</u>

Our original, constitutional energy.
It is the innate energy, before conception, transmitted directly from parents.
The origin, the source of life.
It is the most dynamic manifestation of Jing circulating in the body, in other words, of Qi.
It is the root of all the Yin and Yang energies in the body.
It comes from Prenatal Jing and receives nourishment from Postnatal Jing.
Connected, among the fundamental substances, to Jing, among the Organs, to Kidney (KD) and Triple Burner (TB), and among the meridians, to the 8 Extraordinary Vessels (Mai Qi), which essentially transport this type of energy.
The Yuan Qi that circulates in the Extraordinary Vessels allows the activation of the various Shen in the Organs and the Jing in the Extraordinary Organs.

- It is the dynamic force that drives the functional activity of the internal organs, because, like Jing, it is the foundation of vitality and physical constitution.

- It resides between the two Kidneys, below the navel, in the Ming Men, with whom it shares the task of providing the heat necessary for all the functional activities of the body.

- It acts as an agent of change in the transformation of Zong Qi (Gathering Qi) into Zhen Qi (True Qi). This is how the Kidneys are involved in the production of Qi.

- It facilitates the transformation of Gu Qi (Food Qi) into Blood (Xue) in the Heart. This is how the Kidneys take part in the formation of Blood.

- It dwells, where it originates, between the two Kidneys (at the Gate of Vitality-Ming Men) and relies on the transporting system of the Triple Burner to distribute it to the internal organs and to the meridians. The points where it is most concentrated are at the Source points (Yuan).

GU QI (Food Qi)

It is the first stage in the transformation of food, which is still a raw form of Qi, which cannot be utilised by the body as it is.

It is produced by the Spleen whose function is to transform and transport the various substances extracted from food; it rises to the chest, goes to the Lungs, where it combines with the air, to form Zong Qi (Gathering Qi), a part of which is sent to the Heart, where it is transformed into Blood.

The transformation is aided by the Kidney Qi and by the Yuan Qi.

ZONG QI (Gathering Qi or Chest Qi)

It forms at the centre of the chest through the interaction of Gu Qi (Spleen) with air (Lungs).

It is a finer, more refined form of Qi than Gu Qi, and in this form it can be used by the body.

Its main functions are:

- to nourish Heart and Lungs;

- to enhance and promote the function of the Lungs in controlling the Qi and respiration, and the functions of the Heart of governing the Blood and the blood vessels;

- to regulate the ability to speak and the strength of the voice;

- to act on and promote blood circulation to the extremities.

- it is easily affected by emotional problems such as grief and sadness.

The Zong Qi and the Yuan Qi mutually assist each other: the Zong Qi flows downwards to aid the Kidneys and the Yuan Qi flows upwards to aid respiration (another aspect of mutual assistance between Lung and Kidney).

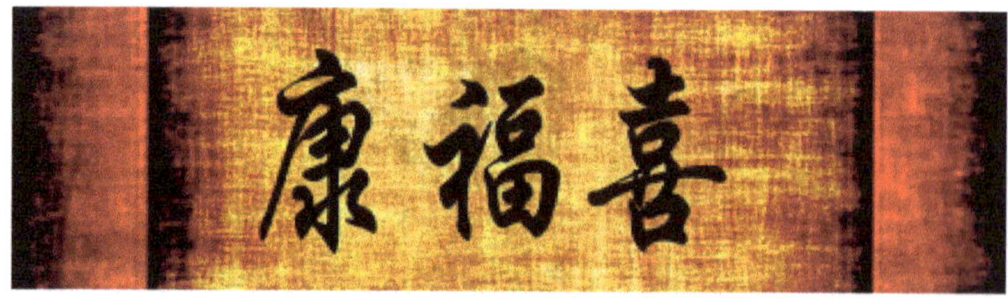

ZHEN QI (True Qi)

It is the final stage in the transformation of Qi.
The Qi that circulates in the meridians and nourishes the organs and viscera.

It originates in the Lungs, like Zong Qi, and adopts two different forms:

- **Ying Qi**

- **Wei Qi**

YING QI (Nourishing Qi)

A more refined energy that flows in the channels and penetrates the inner layers of the body.
It nourishes the internal organs, the viscera and the whole body.
It not only flows in the meridians, but also with Blood in the blood vessels.
It represents a quality of energy that is deeper than the Wei Qi.
It is transported by the Luo Channels and for this reason, it is involved in the more internal disorders, related to emotional factors, digestion and to the organs in general.
Cognitive energy, as opposed to instinctual (Wei Qi), linked to the ability to 'feed on life', and to the choices we make.

WEI QI (Protective Qi)

Instinctual, a more basic type of energy.
It flows primarily in the superficial layers of the body, the skin and muscle, both inside and outside the meridians.
It protects the body against attacks from external pathogenic factors (Wind, Cold, Heat and Dampness).
It warms, moistens and partially nourishes skin and muscles.
It regulates the body temperature through the opening and closing of the pores.
It is conveyed by Tendino-Muscular Meridians (Jin Jing), which represent the most superficial level of the energy structure of the channels (connected therefore to the locomotory system and the immune system).
During the day it stays on the surface, flowing through all the Yang channels but at night it goes deep inside in order to protect Organs and Viscera.
Given that it circulates under the skin, it is under the control of the Lungs, so a weakness in Lung Qi can lead to a weakness in Wei Qi (increasing the risk of contracting illnesses related to the cold).
Wei Qi has its roots in the Kidneys (Lower Burner), it is nourished by Stomach and Spleen (Middle Burner) and is distributed by the Lungs (Upper Burner).
A Wei Qi deficiency can cause a weakening of the body's defences and the person may tend to fall ill and feel cold.

....

The Qi transforms and transports liquids, which would otherwise accumulate and stagnate causing disease.

Qi retains Body Fluids as well as the Blood.

If Qi is deficient it can result in urinary incontinence or enuresis (Kidney Qi Deficiency) or chronic vaginal discharge (Spleen Qi Deficiency).

Body fluids give nourishment to Qi.

After an excessive loss of Liquids, even the Qi becomes deficient (cold hands and feet, pallor, aversion to cold symptoms = Yang Deficiency).

Profuse sweating can also cause a loss of Wei Qi, because it is combined with Liquids that form sweat in the space between the skin and muscles.

"Excessive sweating damages Yang Qi."

"Persistent vomiting causes Qi deficiency"

"Qi deficiency causes sweating"

Body Fluids constantly replenish the Blood and make it fluid so that it does not clot or stagnate.

Likewise, the Blood nourishes and integrates Body Fluids (a loss of fluids over a long period of time can lead to a Blood Deficiency. A chronic loss of blood causes a Body Fluids Deficiency and dryness).

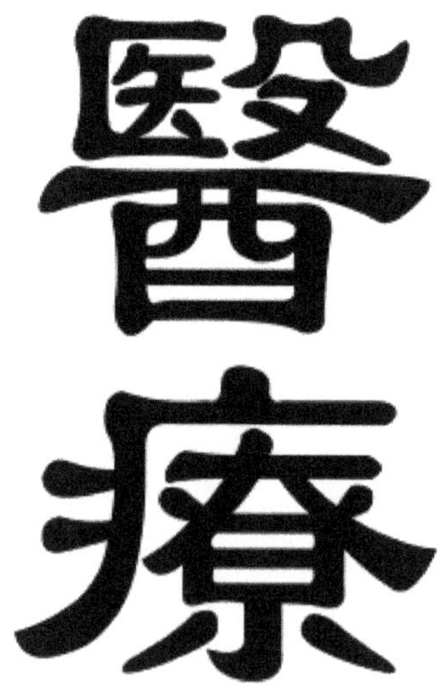

Medical

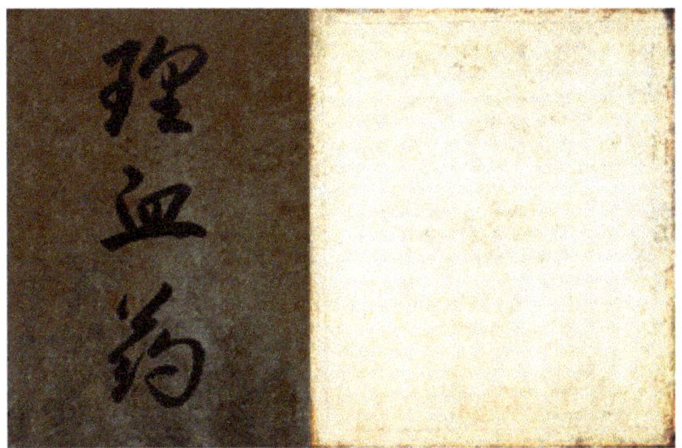

XUE (Blood)

The more material appearance of Qi; more dense, nutritional, Yin.

Blood nourishes the Qi and the Qi moves Blood.

Its main functions are to:

- nourish

- moisten

- establish roots and psychophysical stability

Blood constantly nourishes the bones (during the menopause, due to an overall reduction in Blood available, the development of osteoporosis is facilitated, which is why at this stage in a woman's life it is important to nourish the Blood).

A Blood Deficiency, on the physical level, can result in poor assimilation and excessive thinness, pale complexion, scanty, pale menstruation etc.

Blood derives from food Qi produced by the Spleen and Stomach, which, sent to the Lungs, meets with the air Qi, it is then processed and sent to the Heart, which carries out a final transformation.

The whole process is assisted by the Yuan Qi, resulting in Qi and Blood.

To nourish Blood it is necessary to tonify Spleen and Kidney.

Blood is the material basis for Shen (if Blood is deficient, Shen is without its anchor, becoming unhappy and restless, causing anxiety, irritability, restlessness, insomnia).

JIN-YE (Body Fluids)

The Body Fluids originate from material nourishment (food and beverages).

They are in a continuous process of transformation, therefore the Jin become Ye and the Ye become Jin.

Although divided into Yin and Yang, they represent a very Yin aspect.

JIN (fluids)

They are thinner, lighter body fluids, and they circulate rapidly with the Wei Qi (between the skin and muscles).

They are clear, limpid, like water, and include sweat, tears, nasal mucus, saliva, urine, vaginal and genital secretions.

They are under the control of the Lungs, which help disseminate them to the skin, and of the Upper Burner, which regulates their transformation and movement towards the skin.

Their function is to moisten, nourish, refresh and purify.

They make the Blood more fluid thus preventing its stasis.

YE (Liquids)

More turbid, heavier, denser.

They circulate internally along with the Ying Qi.

They are characterized by a slower movement and find their way to the various body cavities and interstices.

They are joint fluids, cerebrospinal fluid, intracellular and tissue fluids, and serous membrane liquid, etc.

The Spleen and Kidneys control their transformation, while the Middle Burner and the Lower Burner control their movement and excretion.

Their function is to moisten the brain, bone marrow, spinal column and joints.

They also lubricate the orifices of the sense organs (mouth, nose, eyes and ears).

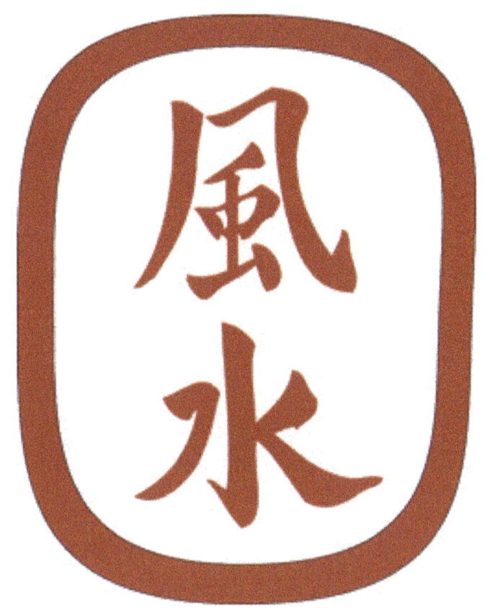

RELATIONSHIP BETWEEN ORGANS AND VITAL SUBSTANCES

The **Lungs** govern Qi and spread Body Fluids.

The **Spleen** governs Food Qi (Gu Qi), regulates Blood and influence Body Fluids.

The **Heart** governs Blood.

The **Kidneys** store the Jing and influence Body Fluids.

The **Liver** stores Blood.

The Organs (Yin) accumulate, store, conserve Vital Substances.

The Viscera (Yang) transform and refine food and drink and extract the purest substances, which are then stored by the organs.

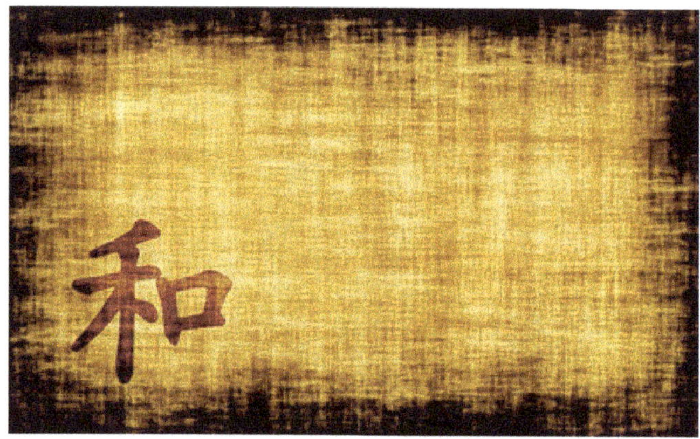

EXTERNAL PATHOGENIC FACTORS

Qi can be transformed from being physiological to being pathological, due to an excess or a weakness in the individual.

Pathogens can enter the body from the outside, just as they can develop internally.

The external pathogenic factors are usually associated with sudden acute illness, while the internal ones are frequently related to chronic diseases.

They enter the body and activate the Wei Qi.

An external pathogenic factor may be:

<u>Strong</u> = eliminated externally (vomiting, sweating, diarrhoea, etc.)

<u>Very weak</u> = going deep inside

<u>Weak</u> = the body is unable to expel it or to internalize it and this leads to a latent pathogenic factor; the body traps, imprisons it, and uses a Yin factor to block the Jing (characterized by an absence of signs and symptoms,) or Blood (characterized by withheld emotions).
As time passes, the Jing declines, is consumed (by age, trauma, etc.), and the body can no longer maintain the latency and as a result autoimmune diseases develop, malignant tumours, diseases that attack the deep level Jing (serious, acute, epidemic illnesses).

The Triple Burner, which transports the Yuan Qi, as do the Extraordinary Channels, is a beneficial meridian to work when treating a patient with an autoimmune disease.

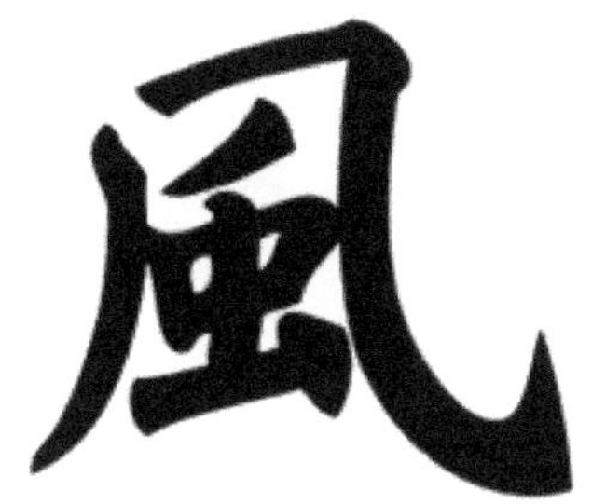

<u>WIND</u>

It is by nature Yang and its characteristic is movement.
It is the most penetrating external factor, and the vehicle of all other pathogens.
It tends to damage Blood and Yin.

The symptoms are similar to its action in nature; here are some examples:

- sudden onset and acute symptoms;
- rapid changes in symptoms;
- shivering, convulsions, paralysis (Internal Wind);
- effects are more intense in the upper and outer body;
- conjunctivitis (External Wind);
- colds, cough, fever (External Wind);
- joint stiffness and pain (External Wind);
- facial paralysis (External Wind).

The External Wind penetrates the skin and interferes with the circulation of Wei Qi, which flows between the skin and the muscles, creating heat. This is why the symptoms are an aversion to the cold.

WIND-COLD

- headache;
- chills, convulsions;
- sneezing, coughing, runny nose, white mucus;
- muscle aches;
- lack of fever or sweating;
- severe pain and stiffness in the occipital area.

WIND-HEAT

- chills, sneezing, cough;
- sore throat, swollen tonsils, itching;
- stuffy nose, yellow mucus;
- fever and sweating;
- pain and occipital stiffness;
- thirst;
- aversion to cold.

WIND-DAMP

This combination that penetrates the skin, over and above the afore mentioned symptoms, causes skin rashes and itching as well as swelling in the joints.

INTERNAL WIND

The main symptoms are tremors, tics, numbness, severe dizziness, seizures and hemiplegia.

Almost always related to a Liver imbalance:

- Liver Wind (high fever, delirium, coma);

- Liver Yang (irritability, headache, severe dizziness);

- Liver Blood deficiency (vertigo, tic, light tremors, numbness, blurred vision).

....

Points for External Wind: GB20 - BL12 - LI4 - ST36 - GV14

Points for Internal Wind: LV3 - LI4 (for facial tics) - BL18 - GV20

HEAT

Yang pathogenic factor (tends to damage the Yin).

Typical effects are:

- aversion to heat;
- sweating;
- scanty and dark urine;
- thirst;
- dry lips;
- pain and symptoms that improve with cold.

Points for Heat: LV2 - LI11 - PC3 - TB6 - BL40

Avoid Moxibustion!

FIRE

It can either be internal or derive from an external pathogenic factor.

Fire may have an effect on the mind (agitation, anxiety, insomnia, delirium, mental illnesses or disorders, etc.).

It can stagnate causing inflammation and ulcers; it can damage Blood and Yin, deplete Qi and dry up Body Fluids.

The points used to treat Fire are the same as for Heat.

COLD

It is a Yin pathogenic factor, so its tendency is to damage the Yang.

It causes stiffness, tightening, tissue contraction, thickening of liquids.

It slows movement and hinders the circulation of Blood and Yang Qi.

It can invade the meridians, causing pain in the joints, tendons and contraction of tendons, chilliness.

It can penetrate organs reducing their effectiveness and activity.

INTERNAL COLD

Yang Deficiency (slowness, hypoactivity).
Often chronic.

> **Excess-Cold** = characterized by the onset of severe and acute pain.
>
> **Cold-Deficiency** = gradual onset of dull pain.

Symptoms vary depending on which organ is most involved:

> **Heart** = chest pain, sense of suffocation, purple lips;
>
> **Spleen** = loose stools, diarrhoea, lack of appetite;
>
> **Kidney** = abundant, clear and frequent urine and back pain, cold feet and knees, impotence, vaginal discharge;
>
> **Lungs** = frequent colds, cough with white sputum.

Points for Cold: ST36 - GV4
Moxibustion is much advised.

<u>DAMPNESS</u>

It is by nature a Yin pathogenic factor, therefore it tends to damage the Yang.

It is associated with Cold and Heat.

It particularly affects the Spleen.

It slows down all functions and movement, creating viscosity, heaviness, inertia.

It moves downward and tends to stagnate, causing pain and constant disturbances, which persist for long periods of time.

It is difficult to eliminate.

The symptoms associated with dampness can be: tiredness, a feeling of heaviness in the head and body, tightness in the chest, cloudy urine, vaginal discharge, loose stools.

EXTERNAL DAMPNESS

Sudden onset of symptoms which are acute.

It can penetrate the meridians causing dull pain and swollen joints (Painful Obstruction Syndrome).

INTERNAL DAMPNESS

Gradual onset of symptoms.

Caused by Spleen Deficiency.

………………………...

Points for Dampness: SP6 - SP9 - ST36 - ST40 - BL20 - BL22 - CV6 - CV9 - CV12

PHLEGM

It forms due to a persistent stagnation of Interior Dampness.

It may take a liquid form or become dense, viscous and heavy (mucus, nodules).

It can also penetrate the meridians (obstructing the flow of Qi) causing swelling and the formation of lumps.

Phlegm in the meridians can also lead to numbness, paralysis and symptoms of mental illness.

It may be associated with other pathogenic factors (Cold Phlegm, Phlegm Fire, etc.)

Points for Phlegm: ST40 - CV9 - CV17

DRYNESS

Being Yang in nature, it tends to damage the Yin and Blood.

It can cause symptoms such as dry throat, mouth, skin and eyes, dry faeces, scanty urine.

Points for Dryness: SP6 - KD3 - KD6 - CV4

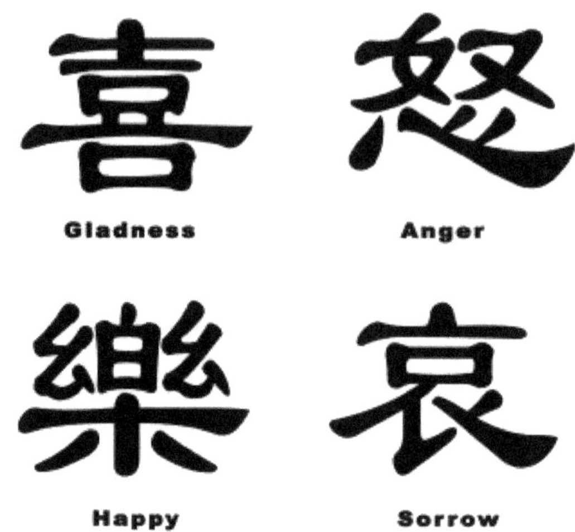

The collection of factors that have a psycho-emotional origin reside in the organs.

An excess or their long-term repression can create imbalance.

They can be both the cause and the consequence of an imbalance.

They each have a specific action on the Qi.

ANGER

It includes different emotional states such as suppressed anger, resentment, irritability, frustration, indignation, rage, animosity and bitterness.

Anger makes Qi rise and it affects the Liver.

It can cause:

- stagnation of Liver Qi (which, over a long period of time, can invade Spleen and Stomach, causing digestive problems);
- stagnation of Liver Blood;
- Liver Yang Rising

Symptoms:

- headache;
- dizziness;

- tinnitus;
- red eyes and sore;
- muscle contractures;
- bitter taste in mouth;
- chronic mental depression (resentment or repressed anger).

JOY

Understood as a state of excessive excitement.

Excessive joy weakens Qi and affects the Heart, through over-stimulation.

SADNESS

Sadness dissolves, scatters, depletes Qi and affects the Lungs (Lung Qi Deficiency).

This condition actually first occurs through the Heart (Heart and Lungs are closely related in the Upper Burner), because it is the Heart that is the first to be weakened by sadness.

Symptoms:

- difficulty breathing;
- tiredness;
- depression;
- crying;
- asthenia;
- amenorrhea (Blood Deficiency).

WORRY

Chronic or excessive worry depletes Spleen and Lung Qi.

It causes stagnation in the Upper Burner (Lungs) and in the Middle Burner (Spleen).

Symptoms:

- shortness of breath, wheezing;
- anxiety;
- neck and shoulder stiffness;
- digestive difficulties;
- blocked diaphragm;
- panic (when also Heart and Kidneys are involved).

<u>OBSESSIVE THOUGHTS (brooding)</u>

Obsessive thoughts weaken the Spleen.

Symptoms:

- lack of appetite;
- asthenia;
- tiredness;
- loose stools;
- phlegm.

<u>FEAR</u>

Fear depletes Qi and damages the Kidneys (by consuming Jing).
It mainly affects the Lower Burner.

Symptoms:

- bedwetting;
- loss of control of the lower orifices;
- night sweats;
- tinnitus;
- dizziness;
- dry mouth.

<u>SHOCK (panic)</u>

Shock disperses Qi and affects Heart and Kidneys.

It blocks the circulation of Qi, causing a sudden depletion of Heart Qi and affecting the Kidneys (the body utilises Jing to make up for the sudden depletion of Qi).

Symptoms:

- palpitations;
- shortness of breath;
- insomnia;
- night sweats;
- tinnitus;
- dizziness.

THE 8 DIAGNOSTIC PRINCIPLES

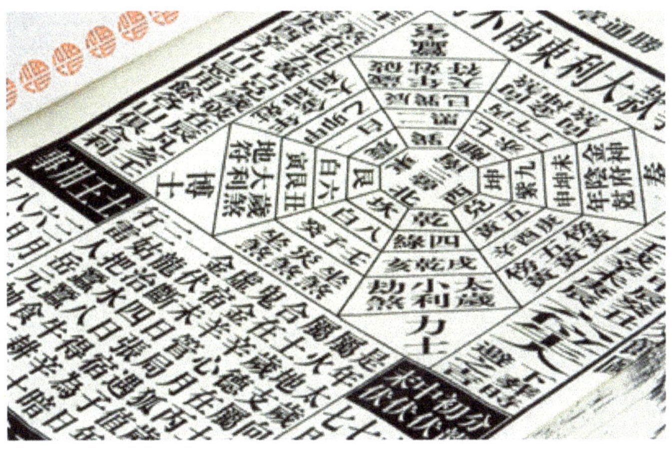

YIN - YANG

INTERNAL - EXTERNAL

EMPTY / DEFICIT - FULL / EXCESS

COLD - HEAT

YIN - YANG

Takes into consideration the general Yin-Yang of the person (physical constitution and energy), the chronic disorders and the acute conditions that are present in that moment.

The Yin Individual: slow, quiet, inhibited, tends to be overweight, sweats a lot even without much exertion, quiet, weak voice, suffers the cold, little body hair but a good head of hair, pale complexion, loves the dark, curls up in bed, weak and shallow breathing, abundant, clear urine, loose stools, long heavy menstruation.

The Yang Individual: active, agitated, lean, outgoing, sociable, loves the light, light sleeper, constipation, tending towards baldness but a lot of body hair, suffers from the heat, hardly ever tired, sleeps stretched out bed, red face, loud voice, talks a lot, breathes deeply, scanty, dark urine, light, short menstruation.

<u>**Yin symptoms:**</u> chronic, gradual onset, evolving slowly, a constant, fixed pain that decreases with movement, heat and pressure, limbs and body cold, pale face, weakness, abundant, clear urine.

<u>**Yang symptoms:**</u> acute, recent, rapid onset, with heat and inflammation, pain changes in intensity, pain moves and modifies, limbs and body warm, red face, restlessness, dark, scanty urine.

INTERNAL - EXTERNAL

An illness can be caused by an external pathogenic factor, which, on penetrating the body (organs), can cause an internal pathological condition.

<u>**Internal syndrome:**</u> an internal imbalance can be generated within the organs, or these organs may have been attacked by external pathogenic factors penetrating deep into the body.
As to the interior of the body (organs, bones and viscera), illness occurs gradually and can easily become chronic, often causing disorders affecting faeces and urine.

<u>**External syndrome:**</u> when an external pathogen attacks the external areas of the body (skin, muscles and meridians).
Acute condition that affects the exterior, often accompanied by a fever and an aversion to the cold, pain, stiffness in the neck. It occurs suddenly and does not last long.

EMPTY / DEFICIENCY - FULL / EXCESS

Refers to the energetic state of the meridians, the Qi, Blood, an organ or viscera.

<u>**Empty syndrome:**</u> chronic illness, weakness, fatigue, apathy, pale face, weak voice, shallow breathing, dull and constant pain that improves with pressure, frequent urination, loose stools, lack of sweating.

<u>**Full syndrome:**</u> acute, severe pain, red face, hyperactivity, restlessness, sweating, strong voice and strong breathing, pain that worsens with pressure, scanty urination, constipation.

COLD - HEAT

Related to the conditions of Full and Empty disorders.

Full-Cold: aversion to cold, pale face, cold limbs, pain that worsens with pressure, desires hot drinks, slowness, clear and abundant urine, loose stools, abdominal pain. It originates from an excess of Yin.

Empty-Cold: cold sensation, dull, pale face, cold limbs, absence of thirst, lethargy, sweating, clear and abundant urine, loose stools. It originates from a Yang deficiency.

Full-Heat: fever, aversion to heat, red eyes and face, thirst, scanty, dark urine, constipation, sweating, burning, excitability.

Empty-Heat: sensation of heat, fever, dry throat and mouth, very hot extremities, scanty, dark urine, dry stools.

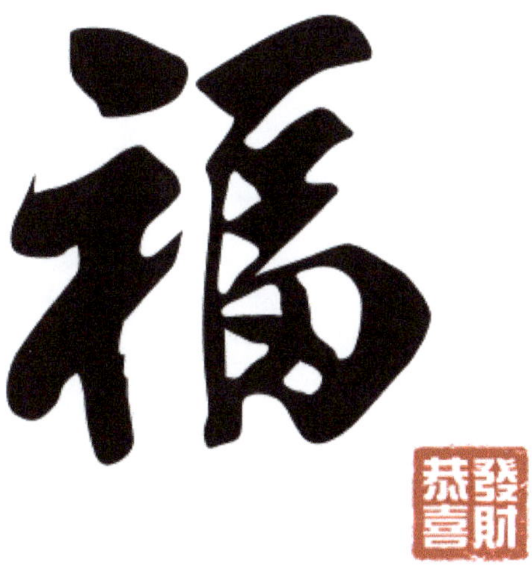

SYNDROMES OF QI, BLOOD AND BODY FLUIDS

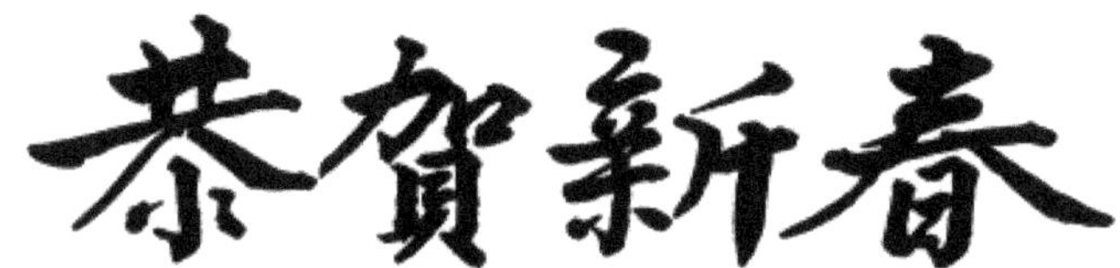

QI SYNDROMES

Stagnation of Qi

It causes a sensation of swelling that may affect various areas of the body and causes a pain to migrate from one side of the body to another or even appear and disappear.

It can also cause irritability, mood swings, depression, sad thoughts and frequent sighs.

Symptoms vary according to the organ concerned.

The Liver is the organ most affected by stagnation of Qi.

Rebellious Qi

When the flow of Qi of a given organ moves in the opposite direction or goes against the physiological one.

This may be due to Deficit or Excess.

The symptoms vary depending on the organ involved.

Lungs = asthma, cough, dyspnoea, etc.

Stomach = nausea, vomiting, belching, hiccups, etc.

Spleen = prolapses, loose stools, bloating, lack of appetite, etc.

Heart = insomnia, mental restlessness, palpitations, etc.

Kidneys = difficulty breathing, coughing, asthma, etc.

Liver = dizziness, irritability, headache, nausea, vomiting, dry stool or loose stools, etc.

Deficient Qi

The most common are the Spleen and Lung Qi deficiency, but other organs may be affected too.

Sinking Qi

An extreme condition of Empty Qi, in which it is important not only to tonify, but also to direct the Qi in an upward direction.

May cause, weakness, fainting, mental depression, prolapse of organs, apathy, etc.

<u>BLOOD SYNDROMES</u>

Blood Stagnation

It can affect various organs, but most commonly the Liver.

Lungs = sensation of chest tightness, phlegm with dark blood, etc.

Stomach= vomit with dark blood, epigastric pain, dark blood in stools, etc.

Heart = sharp chest pain, sensation of tightness, purple lips and tongue, mental restlessness, palpitations, etc.

Liver = abdominal pain, vomiting of blood, painful menstruation with dark blood clots, nails, face and purple lips, etc.

Blood Deficiency

It is often due to Spleen Qi deficiency and Liver and Heart are especially affected.

Heart = insomnia, anxiety, palpitations, poor memory, pale complexion, etc.

Liver = numb limbs, dizziness, insomnia, blurred vision, bewilderment, scanty menstruation or amenorrhea, muscle weakness, cramps, brittle nails, dry skin and hair, pale and dull complexion, etc.

Spleen = asthenia, dizziness, loose stools, numb limbs, lack of appetite, sallow complexion, etc.

Heat in the Blood

The symptoms change according to the affected organ.

It may cause sensations of heat, inflammation, mouth ulcers, skin diseases with red rashes and itching, bleeding, dry mouth, anxiety, mental illness, abundant menstruation, etc.

Blood loss

It can result from Qi deficiency, from Heat in the Blood, from Blood stagnation or Yin deficiency.

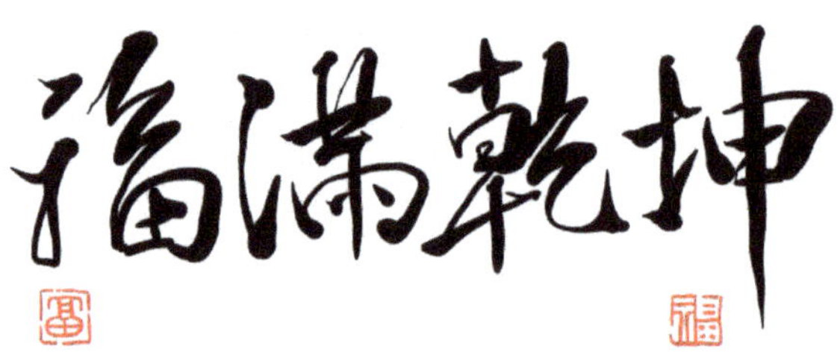

<u>BODY FLUID SYNDROMES</u>

Phlegm

It mainly forms due to Spleen deficiency, but can also be produced by a Lung and Kidney imbalance.

When these organs fail to disperse, transform and expel body fluids, they accumulate and form Phlegm.

Phlegm, in the long-term, becomes pathological and can affect the meridians, internal organs and skin.

There are two types of Phlegm: ' visible' and 'invisible'.

Visible Phlegm = forms in lungs (sputum).

Invisible Phlegm = masses or lumps under the skin (fibroids, enlarged lymph nodes, lipomas), bone deformities (rheumatoid arthritis), Gall Bladder or Kidney stones, numbness of the limbs (when it affects the meridians), mental illness (manic depression, schizophrenia, etc.).

It can take on several aspects:

Wind Phlegm

Stroke, dizziness, numbness, vomiting, cough with sputum, aphasia, etc.

Cold Phlegm

Cold arms and legs, feeling cold in the back, nausea, white, watery mucous, etc.

Phlegm Heat

Red face, dry mouth and lips, yellow sputum, restlessness, etc.

Qi Phlegm

Throat feels as if there is a lump, swelling or constriction in it, hard to swallow, feeling of tightness in the chest, etc.

Damp Phlegm

White, abundant mucous, feeling of tightness in the chest and epigastrium, lack of appetite, lack of thirst, etc.

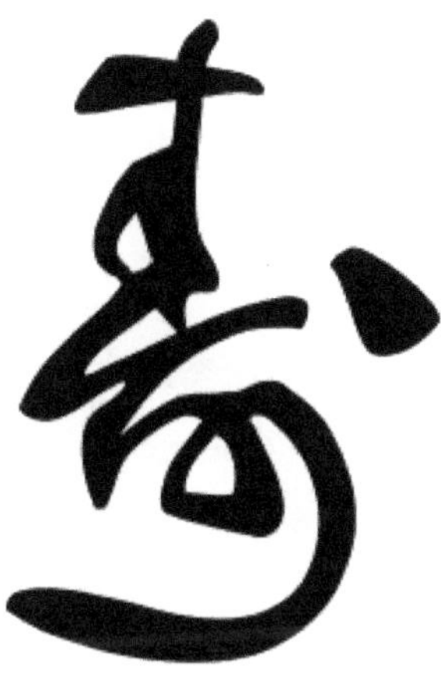

ENERGY NETWORK

A dense network of channels through which the vital energy (Qi) flows.

They carry nutrition to the body (channelling Qi and Blood) and allow communication within the body and with the external environment.

They are divided into two groups: the **JING MAI** and **LUO MAI**

JING MAI Meridians are:

      12 Principal Meridians (Jing Mai)

      12 Divergent or Distinct Meridians (Jing Bie Zheng)

      12 Tendino-Muscular Meridians (Jing Jin)

      8 Extraordinary Vessels (Qi Jing Ba Mai)

LUO MAI are divided into:

      12 Transversal Luo Channels (Heng Luo)

      16 Longitudinal Luo Channels (Bie Luo)

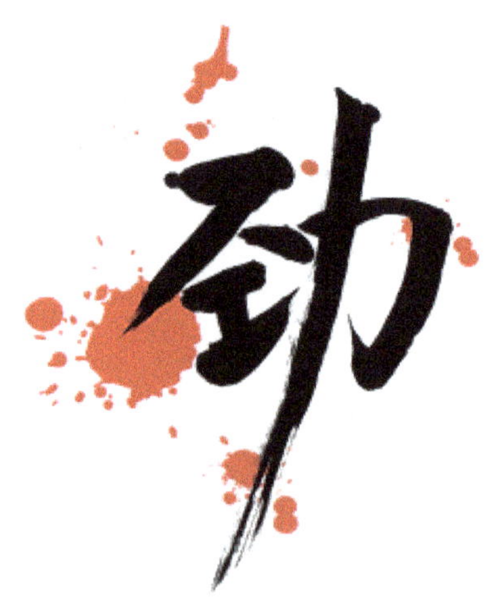

PRINCIPAL MERIDIANS (Jing Mai)

They are formed by the Extraordinary Vessels and become active only after birth; for this reason they are mainly related to the individual's relationship with the outside world and its stimuli (external factors related to climate, social relations etc., and internal factors related to mental and emotional responses).

These meridians govern organs, viscera and the level of energy.

They are divided into 6 Yin meridians (related to the organs) and 6 Yang (related to the viscera) depending on the area of the body in which they flow.

The Yin meridians go from the bottom to the top and the Yang meridians go from top to bottom (viewing the individual with his arms raised), following a symmetrical path on both sides of the body.

Each has its origin in the organ or viscera to which it belongs and represents the connection between depth and the surface.

The connection between the Yang channels takes place at the top and on the surface, while the Yin connects deep within the body.

They are divided into pairs, according to the Element to which they belong (e.g.: Metal = Lung + Large Intestine).

Each meridian reaches its maximum energy activity for two hours in each day.

Mainly Ying Qi (Nourishing Energy) flows along these channels.

DISTINCT or DIVERGENT MERIDIANS (Jing Bie Zheng)

Mainly Wei Qi (Defensive Energy) is transported by these channels.

One of their functions is to connect the Wei Qi (on the surface) with the Yuan Qi (in depth).

These meridians are used to treat autoimmune disorders, joint disorders, complaints that do not seem to have a definite cause and which occur intermittently.

Often it is a weakness of the Wei Qi which fails to ward off external pathogenic factors, and this, in the long term, can deplete the Yang energy.

Their path is deeper than that of the Principal Meridians and even if their tendency is to separate themselves from these, they do, however, have the same name.

They originate from the large joints (knees, shoulders, hips), penetrate deep into the trunk, enter into contact with the corresponding organs and viscera, and all pass via the Heart, finishing in the head ('Windows of Heaven' points and GV20).

Their most important points are all found in lymphatic agglomerations (acting on the immune system).

Distinct Meridians should be treated in pairs, according to the element to which they belong.

TENDINO-MUSCULAR MERIDIANS (Jing Jin)

These channels also take their name from the Principal Meridians and following their path.

They pass through the most superficial areas of the body, and irrigate the muscles.

One of their particular functions is to protect the body from external pathogenic factors because these channels mainly transport Wei Qi (Defensive Energy).

By treating these meridians, you can treat trauma and musculoskeletal disorders, skin diseases, neurological and emotional disorders and acute disorders of the ears, nose and throat.

EXTRAORDINARY VESSELS (Qi Jing Ba Mai)
See specific chapter

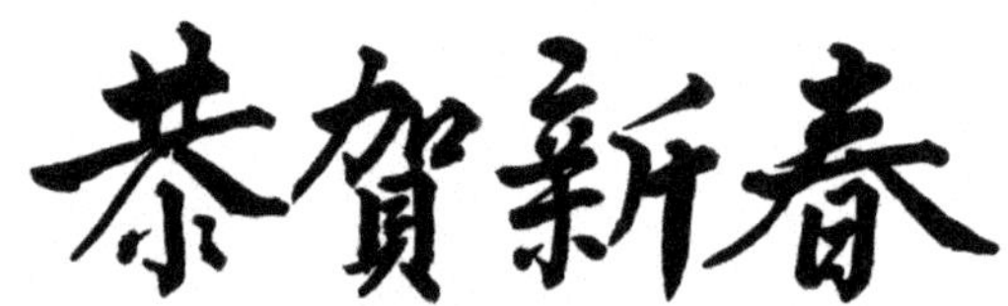

LUO CHANNELS

"Luo Channels, irrigate all parts of the body with Energy and Blood, they nourish the bones, ligaments, and skin and ensure the functioning of the five senses and the six orifices" (Ling Shu – Spiritual Axis).

They form an energy network that connects and nourishes all parts of the body and helps the individual to relate to the external environment.

They never come into direct contact with the organs, as do the Distinct Meridians.

They mainly transport Ying Qi (Nourishing Energy, closely related to Blood) and therefore are often related to internal disorders of an emotional origin.

However, there is an action of mutual support between Ying Qi (Nourishing Energy) and Wei Qi (Defensive Energy) through the Luo Channels. In the case of an invasion of external pathogenic factors, the Ying Qi will support the Wei Qi through the Luo Channels and therefore, in the case of diseases related to internal factors the Wei Qi supports the Yin Qi.

More precisely, these two energies, through the Luo Channels, can be transformed into one another.

They are ramifications that branch off from the Principal Meridians connecting them to each other or to other parts of the body.

They are divided into:

12 Transversal Luo Channels (Luo Heng)

12 Longitudinal Luo Channels (Luo Bie)

and divided still further into three more types of channels which are minute and superficial and which carry nutrients to muscles, bones and skin:

Sun Luo, Fu Luo and Xue Luo

TRANSVERSAL LUO CHANNELS (Heng Luo)

They connect the two Principal Meridians of the same Element.

They start at a Luo point on a Principal Meridian linking it to its coupled partner; therefore they can be used to treat the meridian it belongs to and its partner, including all their anatomical areas.

They create the link between the Wei Qi and the Ying Qi.

LONGITUDINAL LUO CHANNELS (Bie Luo)

Twelve of these follow, more or less, the path of the Principal Meridians to which they belong.

The other four are: Du Mai, Ren Mai, the Great Spleen Luo and Great Stomach Luo.

Since Du Mai and Ren Mai, are respectively the Sea of Yang and Yin, their Luo Channels are used to treat the Yang and Yin of an individual.

SUN LUO

The most minute ramifications. They originate from the Middle Burner and they extend to all extremities, carrying Qi and Blood to muscles and bones.

They generate Fu Luo.

FU LUO

They are the network of tiny capillaries that pass through the uppermost layer of the body, supplying Blood and Qi to the skin.

XUE LUO

These are capillaries under the skin irrigated by Blood. Related to chronic disease with Blood stasis.

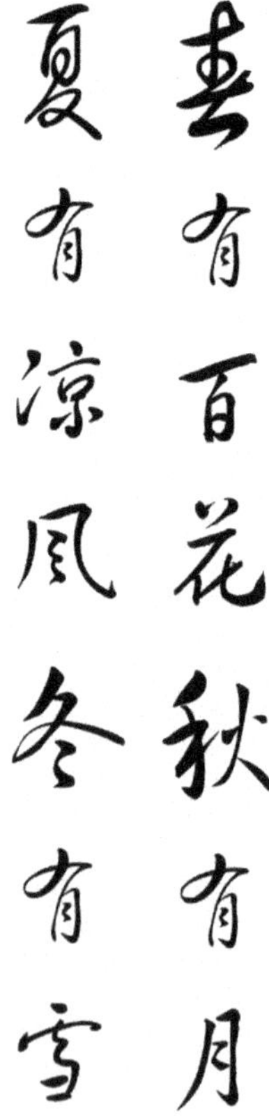

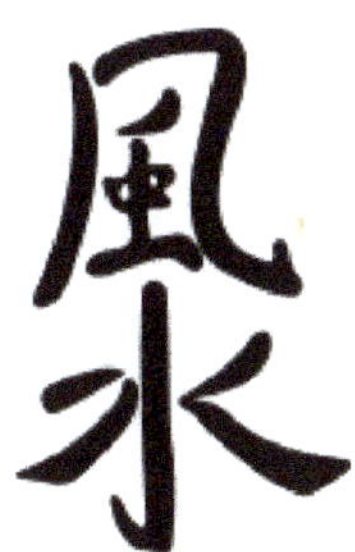

YIN   YANG

YIN		YANG	
TAI YIN	**SHAO YIN**	**TAI YANG**	**SHAO YANG**
LU - SP	**HT - KD**	**SI - BL**	**TB – GB**

ENERGY MATRIX OF THE INDIVIDUAL

=

PRE-HEAVEN

It is from here that the individual begins to live and to do this he needs
to make his way in the world.

JUE YIN	**YANG MING**
PC – LV	**LI - ST**

Bring life to fulfilment. Conclude one phase before starting another. End, exhaustion, death. (LV14 - Qi Meng – Cycle Gate)	Digest life, ability to take from the outside world, elaborate and eliminate.

BEGIN RELATING TO THINGS IN LIFE

=

POST-HEAVEN

77

THE THREE DAN TIENS

DAN = cinnabar, sulphur, mercury, precious substance
TIEN = cultivated field

A place, a field, where something valuable is cultivated.
The three fields, places of transformation, where an alchemical process occurs.

JING - QI - SHEN

The three Bao: the three treasures, the three precious substances.

SHEN (Upper Dan Tien) - in the cranial cavity

IQ (Middle Dan Tien) - in the chest cavity

JING (Lower Dan Tien) - in the pelvic area

JING

Vital essence. The root of the tree of life, something that develops.
The basic material of existence.
One component is transmitted to us by our parents, the other is cosmic.
The capital that life has given us, our energy store.
At the alchemic level it is the raw material, salt.
"The Lead Flower"

QI

Relationship, movement, experience, conflict, overcoming conflict.
"The Silver Flower"

SHEN

Awareness.
"The Golden Flower"

KONG

Emptiness.

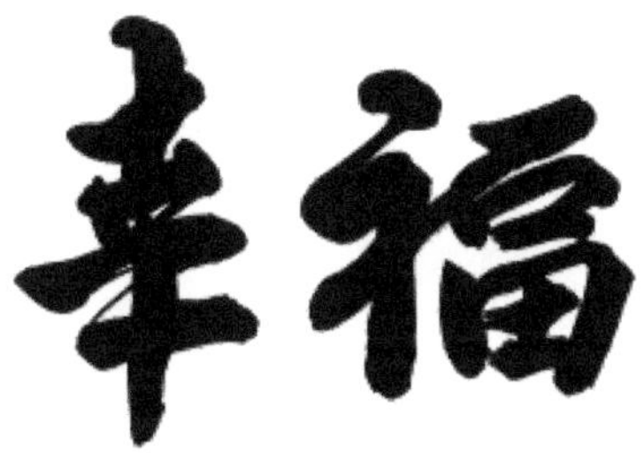

THE SIX EXTRAORDINARY FU VISCERA

They deal with the process of growth and evolution of the individual and of the species.

Uterus (Lower Dan Tien)

GB (Middle Dan Tien)

Brain (Upper Dan Tien)

<u>Marrow - Mai (blood vessels) - Bones:</u> they connect the three Dan Tien with the three Qi Fu (Uterus, GB, Brain).

ZANG (Organs): 'solid', more yin, they preserve and nourish.

FU (Viscera): 'hollow', more yang, they transport, process, eliminate.

QI FU (Extraordinary Viscera)

They do not expel externally.

- They preserve valuable substances (which is the link with the Zang).
- They circulate these substances within the body (this is the link with the Fu).
- They preserve the Yin. Store, modify and nourish.

They are linked to:

- Survival.
- Perpetuation, reproduction (generating new life).
- Spiritual evolution (generating one's own spiritual embryo).

<u>**JIN YE - Body Fluids**</u>

JIN: clear, watery fluids, more yang, moves towards the exterior.

YE: turbid and viscous fluids, denser, more yin, circulates internally (intracellular fluids, hormones, liquor, lymphatic system, etc.). Fluids of the night. They nourish Xue and Jing. They are activated by treating the Extraordinary Vessels.

Both are related to water and therefore to the process of purification through diuresis, sweating, cerebrospinal fluid, blood (through GB).

<u>**GALL BLADDER (GB)**</u>

- Connection between Zang Fu and Qi Fu (several points of the Extraordinary Vessels are on GB meridian).
- Connection between Uterus and Brain.
- Closely linked to the movement of the Ye.
- Involved in all cases where the person avoids or refuses to relate to the outside world.
- Bile is the purest of the Ye fluids, the quintessence.

<u>**QI FU and Aging**</u>

Illnesses related to aging are closely connected to the Extraordinary Fu Viscera (survival of the species, adaptation to radiation, pollution, epidemic viruses, etc.).

Brain	=	dementia, Alzheimer
GB	=	digestive decline
Uterus	=	menopause, infertility, impotence
Vessels	=	arteriosclerosis
Bone	=	osteoporosis, osteoarthritis
Marrow	=	immune system

Lower Dan Tien	Welcomes life	Extinction
Uterus – Jing		

Middle Dan Tien	Relate to the world	Not choosing
GB – Qi	Make choices	Not living

Upper Dan Tien	Understanding life	Not understanding
Brain – Shen	Awareness	"flat encephalogram"

<u>**NAO (Brain)**</u>

Also called 'Mud Pill Palace"
Ability to adapt to change.
Everyone is born pre-programmed by nature.

The brain is connected to:

- spinal column / Zu Tae Yang (BL)
- organs of sense (Qiao) / Zu Yang Ming (ST)

Marrow: Jing+Shen (it is the union between Jing+Shen that allows life to be lived)

Brain: deposit of Jing+Shen - 'Sea of Marrow' - the seat of memory.

<u>Autism:</u>

Lacks the activation of the Middle Dan Tien and therefore the ability to relate; relates only to objects rather than to people.

<u>Brain / Governing Vessel (GV) /spinal column</u>

Hyperstimulation:

- attention deficit
- epilepsy
- allergies (many are caused by hypersensitivity)

Hypostimulation:

- shyness
- demotivation
- down syndrome

The brain, through the Bone Marrow, (via conduction of sensory stimuli) and through the stimulus to change of GB and thanks to the communication process and purification of the Jin-Ye, receives (welcomes) Kidney Jing (Uterus) which is sent out into the world (GB as Qi Fu and Heart as Zang Fu) to become Shen (life experience, self-awareness).

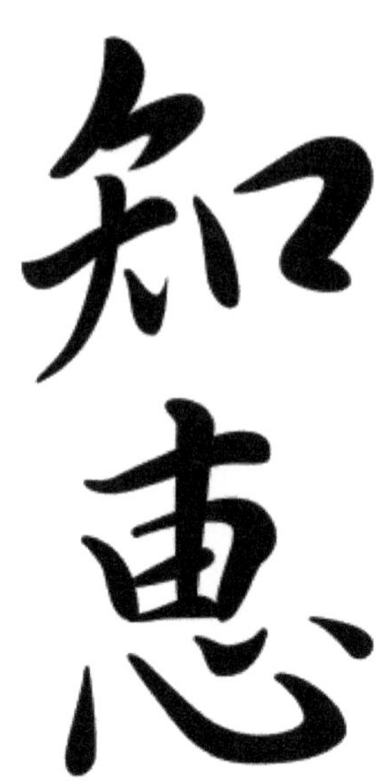

<u>THE 12 PRINCIPLE MERIDIANS AND 3 LEVELS OF EXISTENCE</u>

<u>Level</u>	<u>Function</u>	<u>Channels</u>
SURVIVAL	Breath	LU – LI
Lower Brain	Digest	ST – SP
	Sleep	
	Evacuate	
INTERACTION	Emotions	HT – SI
Middle Brain	Intelligence	BL – KI
	Cardiovascular system	
DIFFERENTIATION	Protection (PC)	PC - TB
Upper brain	Renewal (LV)	GB - LV
	Choices (GB)	
	Habits	

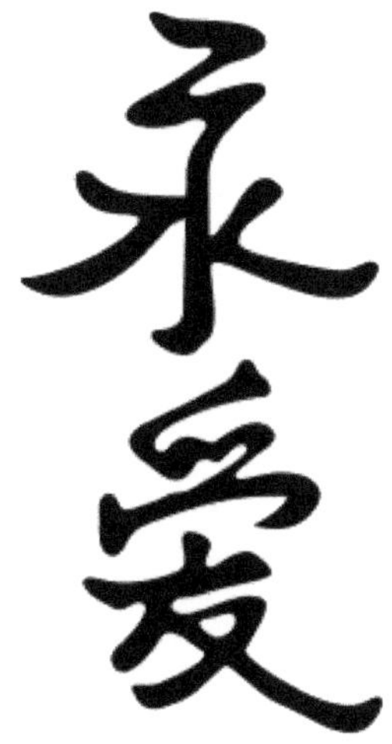

LOWER BRAIN POINTS

GB 20   **FENG CHI – WIND POOL**

Pool: the condition of life
Wind: the wind of change that is brought to the brain

- It brings change to the brain (awareness of self and of the world).

- Connection between GB20 and BL1 (the pressure should be directed towards the corner of the eye on the other side); This connection comes about thanks to Qiao Mai, closely linked to how we see and accept ourselves (Yin Qiao) and how we see and accept the world (Yang Qiao). E.g: a severe case of anorexia, where the person no longer sees herself for what she is- this Lower Brain point can be used (linked to survival) that connects the image (distorted) that the person has of herself (BL1 - Yin Qiao)

- Energetic connection between GB and sphenoid (free to move).

- To bring energy to the head, to increase the capacity to adapt.

GB 11   **TOU QIAO YIN – HEAD ORIFICE YIN**

Qiao means portal and more specifically indicates an alchemical portal; it is the same term used in the Taoist practice to indicate the points that 'open' along the path of the microcosmic orbit.

It is an excellent point to use to free up blockages in the area they are located (head and neck).

The blocked energy in this area can mean:

- goitre
- fibroids
- thyroid
- swollen glands in the neck
- post stroke recovery

It is also used when energy is blocked at the level of GV14, giving rise, for example, to 'the buffalo hump'.

GB11, being a GB point, has also therefore, the function of separating, in the sense of differentiating; it is the point where the Yin enters the ears, and where, amongst other things, it is connected to the Triple Burner channel.

It is a meeting point of TB, BL and SI.

BL 9   YU ZHEN – JADE PILLOW

Bone Marrow Point

It encourages the connection between Jing and Shen.

Having a good connection between Jing and Shen, would mean, for example, being able to sleep well and soundly; good sleep promotes the consolidation of Jing and the recovery of our vital energies.

When we sleep our body grows, it is the Marrow that grows at night and is consolidated; this is because night-time is a Yin period, so, in the absence of the strong daytime Yang presence, all that is Yin can grow and consolidate.

Children grow during the night, so we can help them grow by promoting a state of deep sleep, which consolidates the Jing.

Insomnia can also be viewed as a disturbance in the relationship between Jing and Shen, i.e the communication between Water (Kidney) and Fire (Heart).

Another consequence of insomnia is that the Jing is unable to consolidate itself through rest and quiet, but becomes dispersed because of the continual activity, so that you wake up still feeling tired.

It is also related to the ability to look inside oneself (inner vision can be blurred).

- Aids sleep (insomnia), as it helps the Yin to ascend.
- Specific point for sleep-walking (Yang too active at night, so, the legs move).
- Hot flushes and insomnia related to menopause.
- Insomnia with frequent urination (being a BL point, it favours the ascent of energy, thus preventing excessive urination).
- Stimulates deep and peaceful sleep.

- For mental retardation (as it consolidates Jing at the level of the Brain).
- Growth problems in children.

BL 10   TIAN ZHU – CELESTIAL PILLAR

Supports (pillars) high up (celestial).

- For heaviness in the head (head tends to fall forward).
- It can help the descent of a Yang excess (dizziness from full-heat to the head, mental agitation, dizziness, fainting).
- Excellent point (also BL40) for treating the back (the two points where BL divides into two branches).
- For knee problems.
- Point of the 'Window of Heaven'.
- Divergent meeting point BL /KI.

Thanks to its downward movement action, it helps to move excess Qi, at head level, down to support the Kidney Yang; this involves the passage through the diaphragm, for this reason the treatment of a combination of points which favours the opening and the support of the diaphragm is suggested, such as BL17, CV17 and LU3, to avoid the accumulation of Yang in this area.

GV 16   FENG FU – WIND MANSION

The only GV point through which external pathogenic factors can penetrate.

- Brings the power of change to the brain (see GB20).
- Promotes the ascent of Qi to the head ('brings pure Yang to the Brain').
- Excellent for treating internal Wind (convulsions, epilepsy, restlessness, twitching, itching, etc.) and external (susceptibility to climatic factors).
- Sea of Marrow.

GB 12   WAN GU – COMPLETION BONE
FENG MEN – WIND GATE

- Eliminates both internal and external Wind.
- Connects the head and body (upper body: headache, toothache, mouth paralysis, etc. lower body: weak limbs, little energy, etc.).
- Calms the Shen.

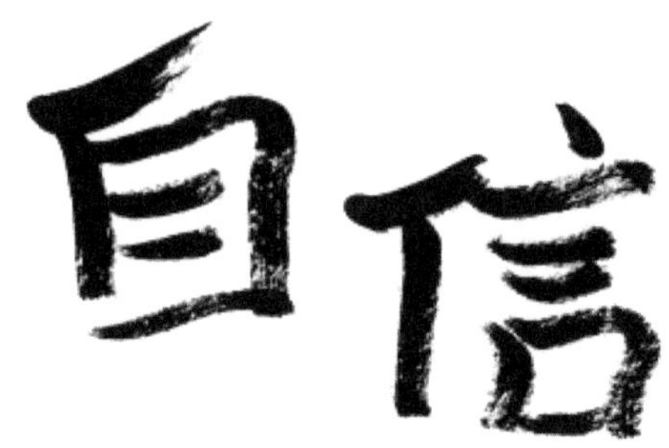

MIDDLE BRAIN POINTS

Communication, relationship with the world and also between the left brain and right brain.

The function of the Middle Brain is to give orientation, a direction to things.

To orientate is also taken to mean making your way in the world, so, for example, circulatory, bone or reproductive problems which are connected to one's own 'circulation', ability to move and interact with the world, are therefore problems that can be treated with Middle Brain points.

The Channels associated with the Middle Brain and that, therefore, can be treated with Middle Brain points, are HT, SI, BL and KD, i.e. Fire and Water.

GV 17 NAO HU – BRAIN'S DOOR

- Promotes the entrance and exit of energy from the brain, invites the Marrow to exit the Brain.
- Point to stimulate memory (brings it to the surface). To bring things out of the brain means to activate and stimulate memory, the ability to remember; stored memories rise to the surface.
- Stimulates a dialogue with the world.

GB 19 NAO KONG - BRAIN HOLLOW (SPACIOUS)

Kong = spacious hollow that follows the Shen

- Provides space, clarity to the brain (for clouded mind, mental confusion, etc.).
- Liberates the Qiao (portals): tinnitus, burning eyes, nose bleeds, etc.

GB 8   SHUAI GU - VALLEY LEAD

The junction point between Lower, Middle and Upper Brain

- For dyslexia (acts on the corpus callosum).
- For people who have one side of the body that is far more dominant than the other.
- For problems of disorientation.
- Stroke recovery, labyrinthitis, etc.
- When there is a beginning of a change that is blocked by the fear of taking risks.
- For Wind-Cold or Phlegm.
  Wind = needs movement
  Cold = blocking action
  Phlegm = stagnation
- Right-left connection.
  Left: active, rational act, governs the right side of the body.
  Right: thoughtful, intuitive, creative, governs the left side of the body.

GV 20   PA HUE - HUNDRED CONVERGENCES

(Also called as NI WAN = MUDDY PELLET)

Junction of Middle and Upper Brain.
Meeting point of all the Yang (all Yang channels converge here).
Strongly connected to Liver (a branch of the Liver channel passes here).
Upper Sea of Marrow point

- Directs the ascent of Yang (prolapse, depression, to revive, haemorrhoids, etc.).
- It also helps to Yang to descend.

BL 7   TONG TIAN – CELESTIAL CONNECTION

On the coronal suture (between frontal bone and parietal bone).
Related to the Brain (GV20), in that the Bladder channel point BL7 goes right to GV20

- Strongly connected to the nose (nasal congestion, chronic sinusitis, etc.).
- Since we are at the level of the Middle Brain, in the case of a blocked left nostril, we will treat the point on the right and vice versa; if both are blocked, we will treat both points. To open the nose means opening the sinuses that are closely related to the head.
- Relationship to the ears (wax in the ears), the Bladder channel has a branch that, from GV20, actually goes to the ears.

– For Phlegm in the brain (confused mind, paralysis, hemiplegia, coma, etc.). Phlegm in the head can also cause a blockage that, however, only affects the area locally, resulting in great mental agitation and, in severe cases, Parkinson (continuous uncontrollable tremors, indicating an excess of Yang, of movement that is, however, circumscribed to the head).

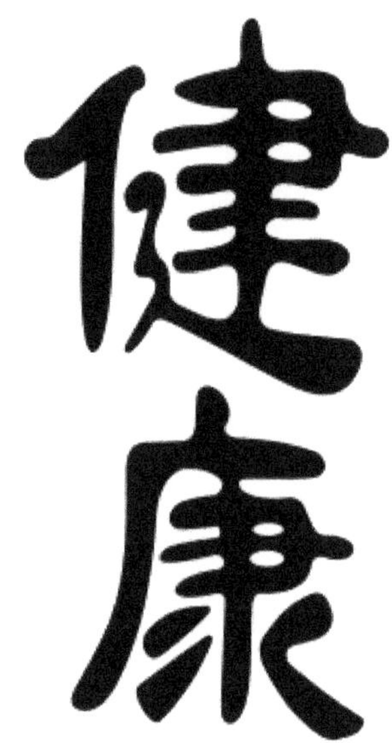

HIGHER BRAIN POINTS

GB 13　　　**BEN SHEN - ROOT SPIRIT**

Wood, Spring, the beginning, require roots.
If the roots (Wood) are solid, Wood can become Fire, Shen, for our evolution.
Ben Shen = where being well rooted (in the world) helps us to understand ourselves.

- For disorientation (where there are no roots).

ST 8　　　**TOU WEI – HEAD CORNER**

Collects life experiences to offer them to the Brain.
Very similar to GB13

- Excellent for detoxification (alcohol, smoking, etc.), with moxibustion.

GB13 and ST8 are involved in the process of individualization which is essential for personal growth.

But individuality also means separation from others.
Often this process of separation from others can also lead to a certain rigidity, therefore, the use of these two points can help the person become less rigid, less stubborn in the way they lead their life.

An excessive sense of separation from others can also lead to an acute sense of loneliness.

These points can also be used to treat people with poor capacity for judgment.

GV 23   SHANG XIN – UPPER STAR

Star = light

Decision making capacity, on both the energetic and psychological level (dizziness, disorientation, etc.).

GV 24   SHEN TING – SPIRIT COURT

It represents the movement (of all qualities of the upper brain) towards the Yin Tang, where all the experiences are collected.

YIN TANG - HALL OF SEAL

Midway between the medial ends of the eyebrows.
The Third Eye.

The dissolution of each experience, the perfect combustion that leaves no residue, the pure fire of Shen.

It represents letting go, abandoning all the experiences of the world that are no longer needed, it is the complete illumination, the no longer having to reincarnate.

This point, however, is not only the dissolution of all experiences, but also the synthesis of all the experiences and memories; therefore, it is a point recommended to treat amnesia (which is the removal of something which, however, is not yet resolved and must therefore be brought to the light of awareness in order to be processed).

All points of the upper brain converge, in one way or another, on this point.

BL 1   JING MING - BRIGHT EYES

The opening of the eyes as in coming into the world.
Linked to the pituitary gland (hormone system).
To move in the world, to choose to open up to the world.
Excellent point for fatigue.

GB 1   TONG ZI LIAO – PUPIL BONE HOLE

Tong = innocence, chastity, purity, new, virgin.

Connected to sight in that it helps us see things with different eyes, always new.
To look at things as if for the first time.
It allows us to be open to new possibilities.

GB = decision, courage, judgement (evaluate)

Deficit = self-condemnation, weighed down by what we have done.
Failing to see the purity that is within ourselves.

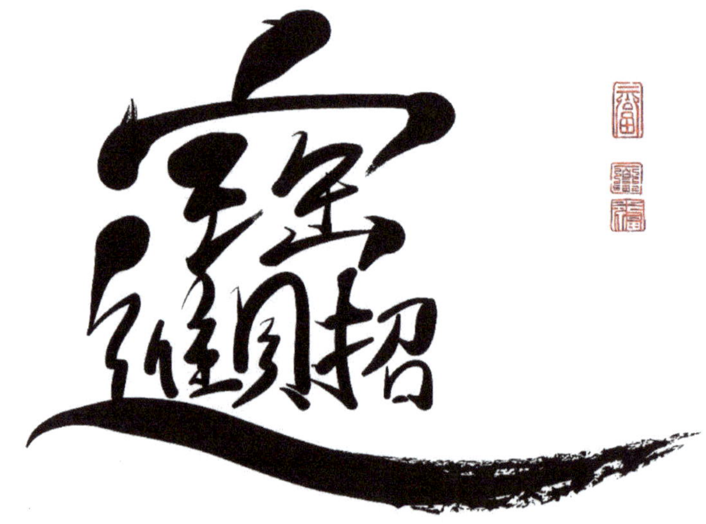

<u>WINDOW OF HEAVEN POINTS</u>

Moving the neck promotes the flow of energy between the head and the body and therefore helps unblock the diaphragm too.

They have a strong connection with the Shen, and therefore have an effect on the psyche.

They collect the influence of Heaven and of the outside world.

They are essentially linked to the Yang channels. Three Yang levels (Wei Qi):

TAE YANG	BL10 – SI16
SHAO YANG	SI17 (GB) - TB16 (in ancient times SI17 was a point on the GB channel)
YANG MING	ST9 – LI18

Superior Line: **SI17 - TB16 - BL10**
Inferior line: **ST9 - LI18 – SI16**

CV 22   TIAN TU – CELESTIAL CHIMNEY

Lowers Qi from the head to the body.

LU 3   TIAN FU – CELESTIAL STOREHOUSE

Supports the Qi mechanism.

'From the chest up is Heaven, from the chest down is the Earth'.

Height of chest = on the arm at the height of the nipple (with the palms of your hands facing outwards).

PC 1   TIAN CHI – CELESTIAL POOL

Supports Xue (Blood).

Location: Externally, next to the nipple.

<u>WINDOW POINTS FOR 'NI QI' (Rebel Qi)</u>

<u>Rebellious Yang (acute symptoms)</u>   **ST 9**

- headache

- fullness in the chest

- difficulty breathing

- lowers blood pressure (even more than BL10)

<u>Loss of voice</u>   **LI18**

<u>Loss of hearing</u>   **TB16**

<u>Spasms and convulsions</u>   **BL10**
<u>Weakness in legs</u>

<u>Internal heat</u>   **LU 3 - TB16**
LV - LU

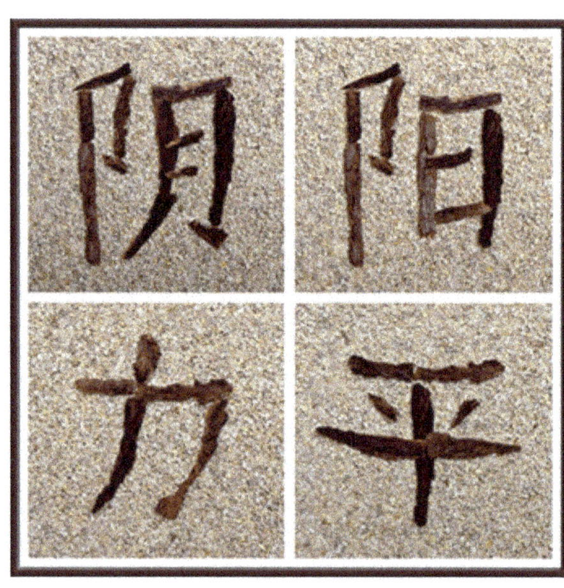

THE 5 SHU POINTS

Also called Transport points, 'Command Points' or 'Element Points' (because each one corresponds to an element).

Five points of each meridian that are located between the fingers and elbows and between the toes and knees.

The energy of these points increases and deepens as it progresses along its path, and its direction is independent from that of the meridian to which the point belongs.

The image is that of a river that springs from a well (fingertips), which flows and flows, deepening and widening until it finally flows into the sea (elbows and knees).

These points are frequently used for their dynamic and effective action.

They are related to seasonal cycles when external pathogenic factors penetrate the body more easily and so can be used to treat these syndromes.

(Jing) WELL POINTS

They are located on the tips of the fingers where the energy flows near to the surface and changes polarity (from Yin to Yang and vice versa).

They are used in acute conditions as they tend to have an immediate and dynamic effect, to disperse and eliminate pathogenic factors.

(Ying) SPRING POINTS

The second point on each meridian, starting from the distal position.

This is where the energy starts to flow faster and with more force.

The action of these points is very rapid, effective and dynamic and for this reason they must be used with care.

As the Spring Points on the feet are the most effective, it is always best to first treat the Spring points on the hands, so as to avoid too intense a reaction.

These points are effective for the release of Heat (febrile illness) from its related meridian or organ.

(Shu) STREAM POINTS

The third most peripheral point of each meridian (with the exception of GB, which is the fourth) and is located near the metatarsals and the metacarpals.

It is in these points that the energy of the meridian starts to flow deeper and with a greater intensity.

External pathogenic factors can enter through these points and penetrate deep into the meridians .

These points are where Wei Qi (Defensive Energy) is collected.

These points are very effective in treating Painful Obstruction Syndromes (especially if caused by Dampness).

Useful for eliminating Wind, Cold and Dampness from the meridians.

(Jing) RIVER POINTS

All the River points are located in the distal third of the lower arm or the lower leg.

On the Yang channels they correspond to the 5th most peripheral point; on the Yin channels, to the 4th point.

Here the energy flows even deeper, with greater strength and breadth.

External pathogenic factors may penetrate at these points and reach various joints, bones and tendons.

They are often used for diseases affecting the respiratory tract.

(He) SEA POINTS

The fifth point, the one located in the elbows or knees.

Here the Qi flows deeply and abundantly, and joins the general circulation of the energy of the body (the river that flows into the sea).

They have a slower and less effective action.

They are used in particular for all illnesses that affect the stomach and intestines.

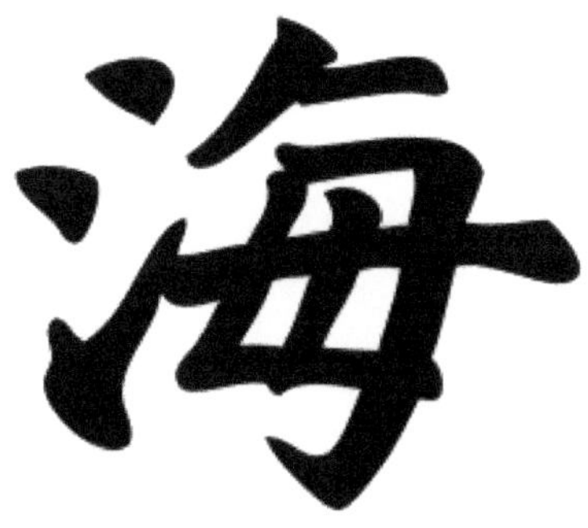

SPECIFIC POINTS

(Yuan) SOURCE POINTS

They act directly on the organs (tonifying) and can also be used in diagnosis.

They are points in which the Yuan Qi (prenatal energy) is most concentrated, closely linked to the organs (especially to the Kidneys) and it is from these points that the Yuan Qi is activated and distributed.

The (Yuan) Source points of the Yin Meridians are used to tonify the organs, while those on the Yang meridians are used to eliminate any pathogenic factors.

(Luo) CONNECTING POINTS

For their action we refer to the 16 Luo channels - 12 Principal Meridians, one for Ren Mai (Conception Vessel), one for Du Mai (Governing Vessel), one for the Luo Channel of the Spleen ('Great Luo') and one for the Luo Channel of the Stomach ('Great Luo').

They can be used alone or combined with Yuan points of the related meridian.

Combining these with the Yuan points serves to strengthen the tonifying action on the organs or the expulsion of the pathogenic factors.

As the Luo Channels are more superficial than the Principal Meridians, Luo points are more often used to treat superficial disorders rather than for internal diseases.

Often it is useful to use the Luo point on the opposite side from where the disorder is manifested, to strengthen the action of the points used on the meridian in question.

BACK SHU POINTS

Qi Entry points

Also known as Transport points, they are treated to directly affect organ activity and to have a strong and rapid effect on their functions.

They are located on either side of the spinal column, along the two parallel branches of the Bladder meridian.

There is one point for each organ and viscera.

The points on the outer branches regulate the mental and emotional aspects of the organs, while those on the inner branches regulate the physiological functions.

They can also be used to act on the sense organ of the corresponding organ.

They can be used diagnostically as they are often painful or particularly sensitive to pressure when their related organ is imbalanced.

They mainly indicate conditions or imbalances that are acute and chronic.

FRONT MU POINTS

Qi exit points.

They are located on the chest and abdomen.

This is where the energy of the related organs and viscera is collected.

Used both in diagnosis and treatment.

These points, too, can be useful indicators of pathologies of the corresponding organs, although not normally used for the main diagnosis.

They are considered 'alarm points' relating to the present state of the organs.

SHU and MU points can be used together to obtain greater and longer-lasting therapeutic effects in cases where treatments are not frequent.

(Xi) CLEFT POINTS

These points are mainly located distal to the major joints of the knee and elbow (except for ST34).

Each meridian has its Xi point (Qi release point).

Used to unblock surface energy and the energy level of the meridian.

They are mainly used for acute conditions, especially for pain.

(Hui) MEETING POINTS

Used for their specific and particular influence on the corresponding Organs, tissues, Blood or Qi:

LV13 for Yin Organs - CV12 for Yang Organs - CV17 for Qi - BL17 for Blood - GB34 for Tendons - LU9 for Arteries and Veins – BL11 for Bones - GB39 for Marrow

THE SIX EXTRAORDINARY FU VISCERA

Brain, Marrow, Bone, Vessels, Gall Bladder, Uterus.

They have an important role, not so much with the treatment of specific disorders, but in the process of individual growth and evolution, described in Taoism as a transformation of Jing, first into Qi and then into Shen.

This process of transformation and purification takes place through the circulation of Jin-Ye (Body Fluids), and in particular the liquor flowing in the Marrow that purifies most specifically the Blood, especially through the action of the Gall Bladder.

The Ye, the denser fluids, are what are mainly secreted by the Extraordinary Viscera, in particular by the Gall Bladder, and transported throughout the body.

Being dense, they flow slowly and, in order to ensure they are abundant and well distributed, the body needs a plentiful supply of Qi.

Cosmic energy, on permeating man, creates three large energy fields: the three Dan Tien.

Communication between these takes place through the spinal column and the Marrow.

- Pelvis = Lower Dan Tien - Uterus - Survival, Jing.

- Chest = Middle Dan Tien - Gall Bladder – inter-relations with the outside world, Qi.

- Skull = Upper Dan Tien - Brain - "Burning the experiences of life"; individual growth, Shen.

They are called the Extraordinary Fu Viscera because their action does not follow the rules that govern other Zang-Fu (the law of the 5 movements, not subject to external influences, not divided into Yin-Yang, not paired to a specific meridian).

They have the characteristics of organs (in that they accumulate the Yin essence and they do not expel) and the shape of the viscera (they are hollow).

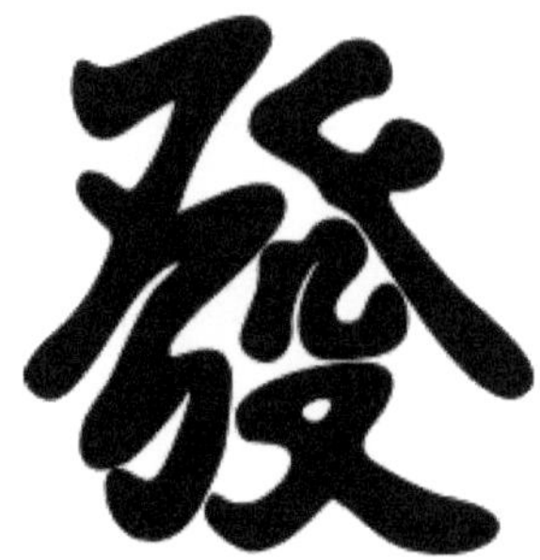

THE BRAIN

The "Sea of Marrow".

Controls memory, concentration, sight, hearing, touch and smell.

Thanks to the conduction pathway of the Marrow and with the transformational drive of the Gall Bladder, it receives Jing from the Kidneys, elaborated until it becomes Shen; the process of individual consciousness.

This action is carried out in harmony with the Heart, where the Shen resides, with the fundamental contribution of the Jin-Ye, which allow its distribution and purification.

Therefore the Brain is closely related to:

- Uterus, as this is linked to Jing and therefore also to Kidney

- Marrow, as a way of distributing Jing

- Heart, in that it houses the Shen

In TCM the Brain is divided into three levels that reflect the three Dan Tien:

<u>1st</u> Level – Survival

Related to the basic functions of man, with all the instinct mechanisms and automatic reflexes.

The physical experience of life (breathing, eating, eliminating, sleep and procreation).

Being rooted to the ground, to life.

The physical counterpart is the medulla oblongata.

At this level the left part of the brain governs the left side of the body and vice versa.

<u>2nd Level — Exchange and interaction with the world</u>

Related to social life, relations with the outside world and therefore to emotions, feelings, moods.

To relate to ourselves, to our ability to observe and analyse our feelings through stimuli and experiences that come from the outside world.

Here, the left part of the brain governs the right side and vice versa.

<u>3rd Level — Learning from the experience of living</u>

Ability to evaluate what one feels, thinks and does, through a process of awareness of one's actions.

And the 'recording' of one's own experiences in order to learn from them and attain personal evolution.

Spiritual growth.

Here, once again, the left part of the brain governs the left side of the body and vice versa.

The connection the Brain has with the Kidneys and the Heart explains how certain symptoms like poor memory and concentration, dizziness and blurred vision, poor hearing and poor vitality may be due to a Sea Marrow deficiency (i.e Kidney) or a Heart Blood deficiency.

THE MARROWS

The term Sui (Marrows) groups together, on the physical level, white spinal cord, yellow marrow and red marrow.

The Marrows link the three major Dan Tien.

Essentially they represent the main means of communication, diffusion and connection between the Lower (Uterus, Jing, pelvis, Earth, etc.) and the Upper (Brain, Shen, skull, Heaven, etc.) but also between internal and external, through the distribution of the Blood that is produced by the bone marrow.

All this happens under the thrusting influence of the Gall Bladder, allowing us to experience social interaction.

They are part of the Ye, dense fluids, deep and full of nutrients.

There is a Yin-Yang relationship between Marrow and Bone: the bone, hard and external (Yang) protects the marrow, soft and internal (Yin) but which at the same time generates and nourishes it.

In TCM the function of Marrow is to nourish the brain, and the spinal column and to produce bone marrow.

Marrow is closely related to the Kidney because it originates from Jing.

THE BONE

The bones have the function of support and protection, not only of the Marrow, but of the whole human body.

The strength and elasticity of the bones are a sign of good Jing and a well rooted Po.

The deep essence of an individual resides in, and is protected by, the Bone.

THE BLOOD VESSELS

They provide not only the pathways by which Qi and Xue can circulate, but also supply the strength that makes this movement possible.

They govern the transformation of Blood, and act as a pathway that carries the Shen to the brain.

Indirectly connected to the Kidneys, because the Jing produces the Marrow that helps to produce the Blood, and the Kidney Yuan Qi also contributes to the transformation of Food Qi and Blood.

THE GALL BLADDER

It is an unusual organ because, unlike the others, it does not distribute, but preserves a precious substance, Bile.

From an energetic point of view, Bile is not only the fluid secreted by the liver that helps the digestive processes, but the quintessence of the seven purifications that food and water undergo in the body.

Bile is the symbol of life, the ability to assimilate, transform, distil and purify all that we take from the outside world.
The Gall Bladder is Fire (Shao Yang together with TB) and Wind (Wood), extremely powerful, mobile and vigorously erect (symbol of the male sex organ); hence its strongly Yang nature.

The ability to powerfully elevate towards Heaven, ability to spiritually elevate oneself.

It is compared to male seminal fluid, to the father figure, who through his example offers guidance.

Sense of deep and interior cleanliness and righteousness.

Linked to the Heart, home of individual consciousness and the ability to discern correctly.

It is located in the Middle Dan Tien, between the Lower, connected to the Uterus, and the Upper, connected to the Brain. It is from here that it finds its ability to activate and move the deep and vital energies, interacting with the outside, allowing us to evolve through a process of awareness.

Hence the link with disorders such as vertigo and dizziness.

The GB expresses, on a spiritual level, our ability to relate to the world, assimilating what it offers and transforming life experiences to provide us with the means to attain personal growth.

THE UTERUS

The deep, vital centre of the human being where creation takes place and the continuous recreation of the individual.

It is linked to the transmission of life and to its maintenance at all levels.

Even in men there is "The Room of Jing". It is a powerful nerve centre connected to all energy structures that are in some way connected to creation; it accumulates and produces sperm and is closely related to the Kidneys and the Du Mai. In fact, if there is a deficiency, the function of production and accumulation of semen by "The Room of Jing" can be compromised and this can cause impotence, premature ejaculation, clear and watery semen, nocturnal emissions, spermatorrhea, etc.

Uterus is:

- The Origin of the 8 Extraordinary Vessels.

- Linked to the Kidneys and to the Jing as sources of creation and life.

- Linked to the Ming Men, the source of organic Yin and Yang.

It represents the crucible where the process of internal alchemy takes place.

We can compare it to the mother and the egg.

Also called "Baby's Bao" due to its connection with menstruation, pregnancy and menopause, the place where 'the inner child' is welcomed but who will then have to grow up and make his way in the world.

Closely related to the Kidneys, the Ren Mai and Chong Mai.

The Ren Mai supplies the Qi and the Chong Mai supplies the Blood to the Uterus; both of which pass through the uterus.

Regular menstruation and pregnancy depend on the condition of the Ren Mai and Chong Mai, which in turn depend on the condition of the Kidneys.

The uterus is closely connected to the Blood in that it requires a plentiful supply at all times and since it is the Heart that governs the Blood, and the Liver accumulates it, and the Spleen controls it, there is a correlation between these three Yin organs.

The Uterus is most closely connected to the Stomach via the Chong Mai (nausea and morning sickness in pregnancy or during menstruation are often caused by influences of the Uterus on the Stomach).

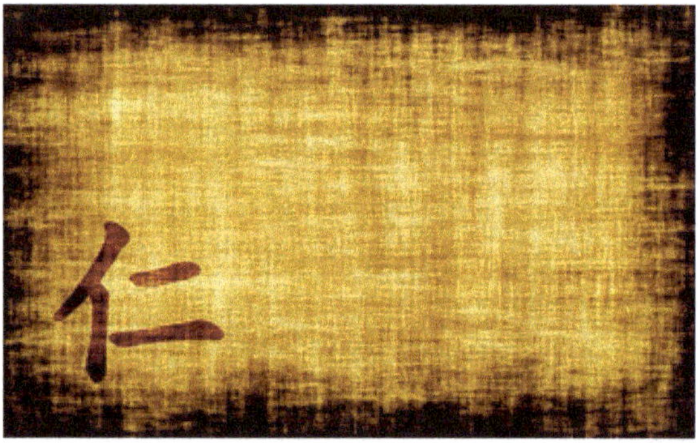

INTERRELATIONSHIP BETWEEN ORGANS

HEART – LUNG

Relationship between Qi and Blood

The Heart governs the Blood and Lungs govern the Qi.

Qi pushes the Blood and Blood nourishes the Qi.

Lung and Heart Qi are often deficient at the same time because of the close relationship that there is between them.

The Heart relies on the Lungs to assist it in moving the Blood in the blood vessels and Lung relies on the Blood from the Heart for its nourishment.

The Zong Qi influences both the functions of the Heart and Lung and the circulation of Qi and Blood.

HEART – LIVER

Relationship with Blood

The Heart governs Blood.

The Liver stores Blood and regulates its volume.

The Heart supports Shen and vitality.

The Liver is responsible for the harmonious flow of emotions.

HEART – KIDNEY

Relationship of mutual support between Fire and Water, and between Shen and Jing

The Heart houses the Shen.

The Kidneys store the Jing.

Heart Fire (Yang) descends to warm Water, and Kidney Water (Yin) rises to nourish Heart Fire.

Shen and Jing nurture each other.

LIVER – SPLEEN

Relationship of mutual support related to Qi

Liver Qi aids Spleen in its functions of transformation, separation and transportation and ensures that the Spleen Qi flows upwards.

It also helps the flow of Bile, an important substance for digestion.

The Spleen helps the Liver to make the Qi flow freely.

LIVER – KIDNEY

Relationship of mutual exchange between Blood and Jing

Liver Blood nourishes and replenishes the Kidney Jing and this contributes to the production of Blood (because Kidney Jing produces bone marrow, which is where blood is produced).

LIVER – LUNGS

Relationship between Blood and Qi

Liver regulates and stores the Blood.

Lungs govern Qi.

Lung Qi helps the Liver to regulate the Blood, and Liver Qi helps Lung to harmoniously circulate the Qi.

SPLEEN – LUNGS

Relationship of mutual assistance related to Qi

Spleen extracts the essence from food and sends it up to the Lungs, where it combines with air, to form the Zong Qi.

Spleen relies on the descending function of Lung Qi to assist in the transportation of food and body fluids.

SPLEEN – KIDNEY

Relationship of mutual nourishment

The Spleen is the root of Post Heaven Qi, while Kidneys are the root of Pre-Heaven Qi.

Post Heaven Qi nourishes Pre-Heaven Qi (with the Qi produced from food) and the Pre-Heaven Qi provides the necessary energy for the digestion and transformation of food (through Ming Men Fire), thus participating in the production of Qi .

In addition, the Spleen and the Kidneys support one another in the transformation and transportation of body fluids.

LUNGS – KIDNEYS

Relationship of Qi and Fluids

Lungs govern the Qi and respiration and send Qi down to the Kidneys where it is held.

Lungs control the water passages and push Fluids down to the Kidneys, which in turn respond by evaporating some of the Fluids, sending this vapour back to the Lungs to keep them moist.

SPLEEN – HEART

Relationship with Blood

Both have a connection with Blood.

The Spleen produces the Blood and the Heart governs it and moves it along the blood vessels (which the Spleen controls).

If the Spleen fails to produce enough Blood (Deficient Spleen Qi), this will inevitably lead to a Heart Blood Deficiency (dizziness, palpitations, poor memory, insomnia, etc.).

If the Heart cannot pump the Blood to the vessels (Heart Yang Deficiency), the Spleen function of production and control of Blood will be impaired.

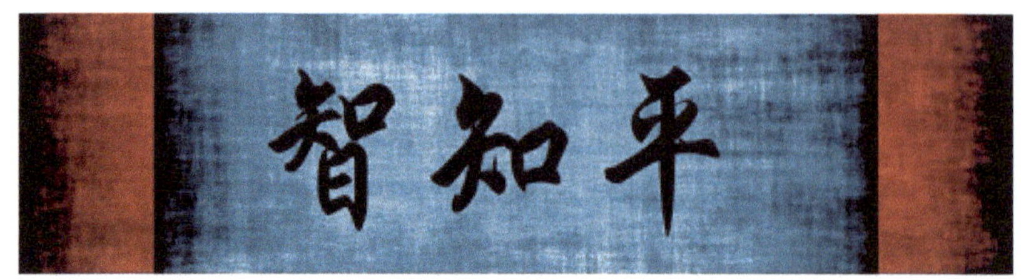

LUNG

EXCHANGE

SHU POINT = BL13   **MU POINT = LU1**

03:00 to 05:00 a.m.

DISPERSION
EXCHANGE
RESPIRATORY SYSTEM
ENTRY AND EXIT (in the stages of life, emotional and affective sphere)
BIRTH / DEATH
LIMITS, BOUNDARY, FRONTIER
PROTECTION
EXTERNAL RELATIONSHIPS
ANTISOCIAL BEHAVIOUR
LEARNING (experiential)
MEMORY (PO) - GENETICS (INSTINCT), CORPOREAL, PAST LIVES
REPETITIVE BEHAVIOUR (PHYSICAL AND PSYCHOLOGICAL)
CAPACITY OF INTROSPECTION
RETENTION
PAIN
TEARS
SADNESS
DEPRESSION
MOURNING
SKIN
BODY HAIR

"The Prime Minister on whom the rhythmic order depends."

"The Receiver of heavenly Qi"

<u>**FUNCTIONS**</u>

- Govern Qi and respiration.

- Regulate the exchange with the outside and internal order.

- Supply the Blood with oxygen, eliminating carbon dioxide.

- Lower and diffuse Qi.

- Assimilates the pure Qi from the air and from the sun (through the skin), which combines with the food Qi that comes from the Spleen to form the Zong Qi, which is sent to every part of the body to nourish all the tissues and support all physiological processes.

- Regulate the circulation in both the meridians and blood vessels, spreading Qi throughout the body and the Blood through the vessels so it can nourish, moisten and warm the body.

- Spread the Wei Qi and body fluids throughout the body, in the space between the skin and muscle, to protect the body from external pathogenic factors.

- Regulate and move the Water Passages.

- Direct Qi and Body Liquids downwards (towards Kidneys and Bladder).

- Control the expulsion of some of the body fluids through sweating.

- Cool and purify the body through sweating.

- Govern skin and body hair.

- Open into the nose and govern the voice (tone, strength, clarity) - "The Lungs have their door in the throat and they house the vocal cords."

- House the Po (corporeal soul): genetic memory of the processes of the species (instinct), corporeal memory of the experiences acquired in the life, the memory of past lives.

- Ability to relate to others and to relate to one's inner self.

<u>**DISORDERS / DYSFUNCTIONS**</u>

- Stagnation of Qi in upper region of body (cough, shortness of breath, chest tightness, constipation).

- Stagnation of fluids in upper region of body (face oedema, dry skin, abnormal urination, swollen and watery eyes, nasal congestion).

-   Invasion of External <u>Wind</u> (weak Wei Qi) (hoarseness, aphonia, etc.), <u>Cold</u> (chills, lack of sweating, cold, acute or chronic bronchitis, bronchial asthma, emphysema, cough with watery sputum, etc.), <u>Heat</u> (fever, chills, sweating, thirst, constipation, inflamed, swollen and painful throat, asthma or a cough with yellow, sticky sputum, thick, yellow nasal mucous, dry nose and nasal bleeding, etc.), <u>Dampness</u> (bronchitis or bronchial asthma with white mucous - Cold - or yellow mucous – Heat).

-   Skin problems (chronic diseases such as eczema or psoriasis, dry and pale skin, redness and burning = internal disturbance, usually from Blood Heat).

-   Yin and Lung Qi deficiency (pulmonary tuberculosis, chronic pharyngitis, bronchitis, chronic cough with almost no sputum, blood in the sputum, quiet voice, afternoon fever, night sweats, fatigue, dyspnoea and weak voice, etc.).

-   Cold limbs (especially the hands): weak Lung Qi, not able to move the blood.

-   Constipation (weak Lung Qi that does not assist with peristalsis).

-   Urinary retention, especially in the elderly.

-   Emotional problems, grief, depression, sadness, pain, anxiety, etc.

-   Dyspnoea (food stagnation and chronic constipation).

-   Depressive syndromes (Lung Qi stagnation), usually combined with chronic constipation.

-   Poor respiration which leads to poor blood circulation, loss of vigour, depression, mental and physical exhaustion.

LUNG QI DEFICIENCY

Cough, rhinitis, dyspnoea, asthenia, daytime sweating, aversion to cold, shortness of breath and shallow, weak voice, dizziness, sputum and clear fluid, etc.

<u>Causes:</u>
Hereditary predisposition; sedentary lifestyle; invasion of External Wind-Heat or Wind-Cold invasions.

LUNG YIN DEFICIENCY

Dry cough, hoarse voice, aphonia, thick catarrh, possibly blood tinged, dry mouth and/or throat, evening fever, red cheeks, night sweats, etc.

<u>Causes:</u>
Long term Lung Qi deficiency; excessive fatigue; chronic cough; presence of Fire that causes Body Fluid deficiency; Stomach Yin deficiency (irregular eating habits, eating in a hurry).

LUNG DRYNESS

Dry cough, sticky sputum, low, husky voice, aphonia, dry mouth and throat, thirst, dry skin, etc.

Causes:

External invasion; presence of Wind-Heat that consumes Body Fluids; Stomach Yin deficiency (incorrect and irregular diet, worries, etc.).

DAMP-PHLEGM OBSTRUCTING

Cough with profuse, white sputum, fullness of the chest, shortness of breath, nausea, loss of appetite, etc.

Causes:

Invasion of External Wind-Cold and Dampness; Spleen Deficiency; excessive consumption of fatty and / or raw foods.

PHLEGM-HEAT OBSTRUCTING

Dry, barking cough, abundant, smelly, dark/green sputum, shortness of breath, asthma, tightness in chest, etc.

Causes:

Excessive alcohol consumption, smoking, fatty foods, spicy, etc.

WIND-COLD INVASION

Cough with white, fluid sputum, nasal congestion, sneezing, aversion to cold, chills and fever, muscle aches, etc.

Causes:

Invasion of external Wind-Cold; particular weakness of all types of body Qi.

WIND-HEAT INVASION

Cough with yellow sputum, fever, sore throat, stuffy nose, headache, aching muscles, slight sweating, etc.

Causes:

Invasion of external Wind and Heat.

LUNG MERIDIAN POINTS

LU 1   ZHONG FU – CENTRAL STOREHOUSE

Mu point for Lung
Meeting point of Tai Yin (LU – SP)

- Regulates Lung Qi and calms coughs.

- Stimulates the descent of Lung Qi.

- Disperses fullness of the chest (Full Lung) and blocks acute pain syndromes.

- Cools Heat in the Lungs (when an external pathogenic factor has already penetrated the body).

- Together with ST40 transforms Phlegm retained in the chest.

- Effective for shoulder or upper back pain caused by dysfunction of the Lung meridian.

- As well as BL13, LU1 tonifies the Lungs or eliminates both acute and chronic pathogenic factors.

- As well as ST36 and SP3, LU1 tonifies Spleen and Lungs: "Nurture the Earth to generate Metal."

LU 2   MEN YUN – CLOUD GATE

Same actions as LU1

- Eliminates excess Lung Qi

- Stimulates the descent of Lung Qi.

- Calms coughs.

LU 3   TIAN FU – CELESTIAL STOREHOUSE

- Powerful effect on problems of an emotional nature (deep sadness, depression, great distress, claustrophobia, agoraphobia, mental confusion and memory loss, etc.).

LU 4   BAI XIAN – GUARDING WHITE

-   Transforms Phlegm and drains Damp from the Middle Burner.

LU 5   CHI ZE – CUBIT MARSH

(He) Sea point, (also known as Uniting Point) corresponding to the Water phase (as it is on a Yin channel).
Dispersion point

-   Stimulates descending of Lung Qi.

-   Cools Heat in the Lungs (cough, fever, thirst and yellow sputum).

-   Disperses Lung Phlegm (chronic bronchitis: with ST40 - pertussis: with LU10 and ST40).

-   With KI7 to cleanse the Lungs and nourish Yin.

-   Helps the Bladder, since it opens the Water passages (urine retention caused by obstruction of the Lungs due to Damp-Phlegm, which prevents the Lung Qi from descending to the Kidneys - with SP9 and CV3).

-   Relaxes the tendons of the arm (Painful Obstruction Syndrome of the elbow caused by invasion of Wind and for cases where the person is unable to lift the arm).

LU 6   KONG ZUI – COLLECTION HOLE

(Xi) Cleft point

-   Regulates Lung Qi and stimulates the descent of Lung Qi to the Middle Burner and to Kidneys.

-   Cools Heat.

-   Controls bleeding (Xi point).

-   Effective in acute, Full Lung syndromes, especially for acute asthma.

-   Tonifies Heart Qi, in the case of a Deficiency caused by deep sadness.

-   Calms the Shen.

LU 7   LIE QUE – BROKEN SEQUENCE

(Luo) Connecting point for Lung and Large Intestine channels
Master point of CV

- Circulates defensive energy, the Wei Qi, thus releasing the exterior (Wind-Cold or Wind-Heat) – paired with LI4.

- Effective point for eliminating pathogenic factors, as it stimulates the descent and circulation of Lung Qi, releasing the Wei Qi and promoting perspiration (also for all types of acute and chronic cough and asthma).

- In the early stages of a cold or flu (sneezing, runny nose, stuffy nose, stiff neck, headache, cold, etc.) - paired with LI20.

- One of the most important and effective points for its effect on the face and head (headaches).

- It can have a noticeable effect on the psyche (emotional problems: worry, sadness or distress, moods and repressed emotions, restrained tears).

- Calms the Shen and promotes a residence to Po (releasing tension in the chest).

- Distal point for Painful Obstruction Syndrome of the shoulder.

- Paired with KI6 facilitates the descent of Lung Qi and helps Kidneys to carry out their function of storing Qi (asthma, chronic Lung and Kidney Deficiency, facial oedema).

- Paired with KI6 tonifies the Yin (regulates the uterus and the menstrual cycle).

- As this is the Lung point that regulates the Water passages, it is indicated for all cases of retention (oedema, urinary retention).

- Can be used to treat milk let-down difficulties during lactation.

LU 8   JING QU - CHANNEL DITCH

(Jing) River point, corresponding to Metal phase

- Effective for ailments in the throat and lungs, cough and asthma.

LU 9   TAI YUAN – GREAT ABYSS

Stream point, corresponding to Earth phase
(Yuan) Source point
(Hui) Meeting point of arteries and veins
Tonification point

- Tonifies Lung Qi and Yin, especially in chronic diseases.

- Eliminates Phlegm from the Lungs (chronic cough with yellow, sticky sputum).

- Tonifies the Zong Qi (in cases of Qi deficiency: cold hands and weak voice) – paired with CV17.

- Affects all blood vessels (poor circulation, cold hands and feet, chilblains and varicose veins).

- Stimulates the circulation of Heart Qi and Blood in the chest (exertional dyspnoea, palpitations).

- Clears Lung and Liver Heat.

LU 7	LU 9
External issues, Excess syndromes	Internal issues, Deficiency syndromes
Releases to the Exterior	Releases to the Interior
Acts on the Qi	Acts on Qi and Blood
Indicated for meridian problems	Not suitable for meridian problems
More suitable for emotional problems	Less suitable for emotional problems
Does not dissolve Phlegm	Dissolves Phlegm
Opens Water passages	Does not open Water passages

LU 10   YU JI - FISH BORDER

(Ying) Spring point, belonging to the Fire phase.

- Cools Heat in Lungs, especially in acute situations.

- Improves conditions of the throat (clears Heat).

LU 11   SHAO SHANG – LESSER SHANG

(Jing) Well point, corresponding to Wood phase.

- Clears External Wind Heat (sore throat).

- Promotes the descent and diffusion of Lung Qi.

- Effectively clears Internal Wind (along with other Well points on the hand, the loss of consciousness that occurs in a cerebra-vascular attack, opens the orifices and revives after fainting).

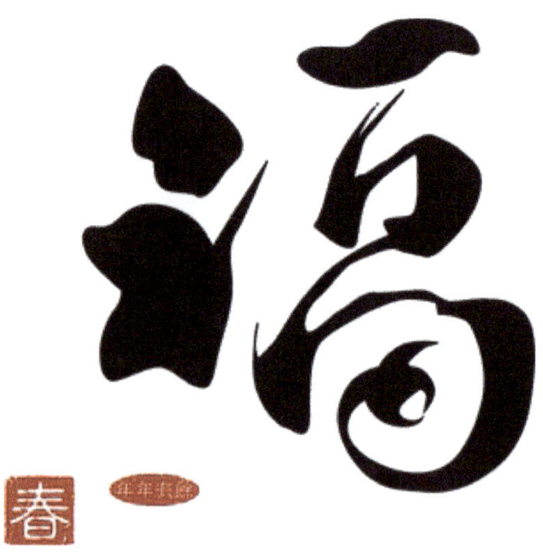

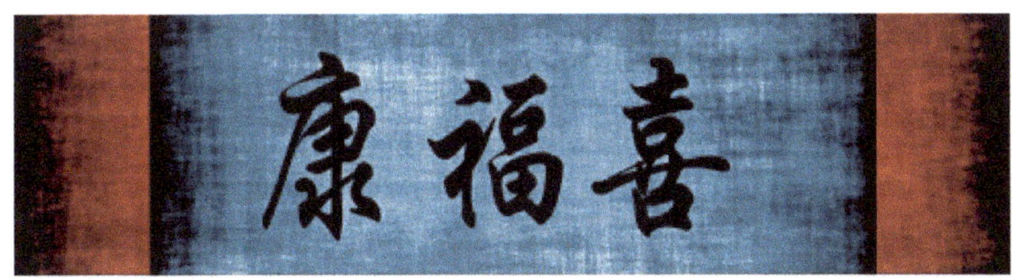

LARGE INTESTINE

ELIMINATION

SHU POINT = BL25   **MU POINT = ST25**

5:00 to 07:00 a.m.

RELATIONSHIP WITH THE OUTSIDE WORLD
RETENTION (eg constipation, but also in the material sense, eg hoarding)
PAIN
SADNESS
TEARS
DISSATISFACTION
COMPLAIN
EMOTIONAL STABILITY
NEGATIVE ATTITUDE
NARROW MINDEDNESS
INFLEXIBILITY
PLAINTIVE VOICE

The origin of evolution and change.

FUNCTIONS

- Receives food from the Small Intestine, absorb fluids, and excretes the remainder in faeces.

- Constipation (stagnation of Lung Qi).

- Sinusitis, common colds or hay fever.

- Acne, pimples, blisters.

- Feeling cold, poor circulation in the lower Hara (uterus, ovaries, bladder, intestines, lower back region) and in the legs.

- Stagnation (inability to let go).

- Perennial dissatisfaction, depression, emotional closure.

- Feeling of abdominal bloating.

- Headache.

HEAT

Constipation, dry stools, scanty, dark urine, pain and burning in anus, burning in the mouth, etc.

<u>Causes:</u>
Excessive consumption of hot and dry food.

DAMPNESS-HEAT

Abdominal pain, pain and burning in anus, diarrhoea, stools with blood and mucus, scanty, dark urine, fever, sweating, thirst, dry mouth, tightness in the chest, heaviness, etc.

<u>Causes:</u>
Emotional (worry, anxiety, etc.).

DRYNESS

Ascent of impure Qi, obstinate constipation with dry stools that are difficult to evacuate, dry mouth and throat, dizziness, etc.

<u>Causes:</u>
General dehydration of the body; excess External Heat; Blood or Yin deficiency; failure of Stomach fluids to descend.

COLD

Abdominal pain, chills, diarrhoea, bowel sounds, pale urine, etc.

Causes:
External Cold invasion; excessive consumption of cold foods.

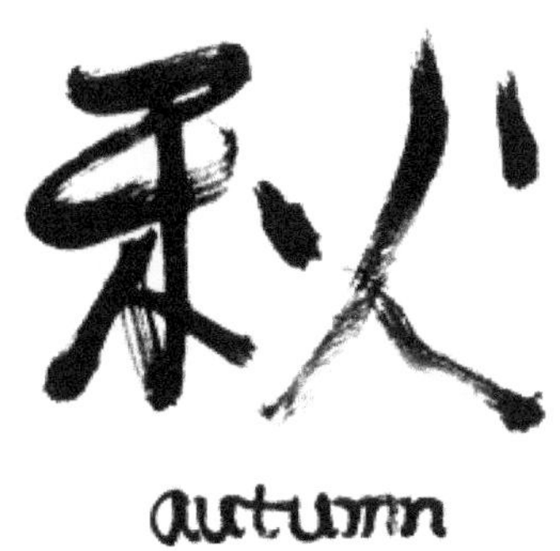

LARGE INTESTINE MERIDIAN POINTS

LI 1   **SHANG YANG – METAL YANG**

(Jing) Well point, corresponding to Metal phase

- Rapidly removes blockages in cases of Excess Syndromes.

- Clears Heat (Internal and External).

- Useful for eye conditions caused by External Wind-Heat (acute conjunctivitis).

- Expels Wind and Cold from the meridian (Painful Obstruction Syndrome of the shoulder).

- Calms the Shen.

LI 2   **ER JIAN - SECOND SPACE**

(Ying) Spring point, corresponding to Water phase.
Sedation point

- Clears Heat from the LI (constipation, dry stool, fever and abdominal pain).

LI 3   SAN JIAN - THIRD SPACE

(Shu) Stream point, corresponding to Wood phase.

- Expels External Wind in the Painful Obstruction Syndrome of the hand (Stream points are recommended for the treatment of joint pain).

- Expels Wind-Heat (illuminates the eyes and is beneficial to the throat).

LI 4   HE GU - UNION VALLEY (GREAT ELIMINATOR)

(Yuan) Source point

- Expels Wind-Heat and releases the Exterior (nasal congestion, sneezing, cough, stiff neck, allergic rhinitis, sore eyes, etc.).

- Removes obstructions from the meridian (Painful Obstruction Syndrome of the arm or shoulder).

- Strengthens and circulates Lung Qi.

- Any problem of the face, mouth, nose, eyes (allergic rhinitis, conjunctivitis, mouth ulcers, sties, sinusitis, epistaxis, toothache, trigeminal neuralgia, facial paralysis, headache with pain on forehead, etc.).

- Paired with LV3 ('The Four Gates') to expel Internal or External Wind from the head, stop pain and calm the Shen.

- Paired with KD7 influences perspiration (reduce or stimulate).

- Paired with ST36 and CV6 for chronic allergic rhinitis (treatment to be carried out between attacks).

- Harmonizes the ascent of Yang and the descent of Yin (in cases of Rebel Qi - Stomach, Lung, and Liver Qi rebelling upwards and Spleen Qi sinking).

- Promotes the start of labour (not advisable during pregnancy, especially in the first three months).

LI 5   YANG XI – YANG RAVINE

(Jing) River point, corresponding to Fire phase.

- Expels Wind-Heat and releases the Exterior in the early stages of invasion by External Pathogenic Factors.

- For Painful Obstruction Syndrome in the hand and wrist.

LI 6   PIAN LI – VEERING PASSAGEWAY

(Luo) Connecting point of the Large Intestine channel and its complimentary channel, Lung.

- Regulates Lung Water passages (oedema of the face and hands, chronic conditions of Lung Qi Deficiency).
- Very effective for mental conditions (manic depression).

LI 7   WEN LIU – WARM DWELLING

(Xi) Cleft point

- Alleviates pain.
- Removes obstructions from the meridian (acute conditions).
- Expels External Wind-Heat (sore throat or swollen tonsils).

LI 8   XIA LIAN - LOWER RIDGE

- Eases pain.
- Expels Wind, Phlegm and Dampness.

LI 9   SHANG LIAN – UPPER RIDGE

- Expels Wind-Damp and clears Heat.

LI 10   SHOU SAN LI - ARM THREE LI

- Powerful Qi and Blood tonic.
- Removes obstructions from the meridian (for all the problems of the LI meridian).
- For any muscular problem of the forearm and hand.

LI 11   QU CHI – POOL AT THE BEND

(He) Sea point, corresponding to Earth phase.
Tonification point

- Expels external Wind-Heat (invasions with fever, cold, stiff neck, sweating, runny nose and an aching body). Not specifically for the face as is LI4.

- Clears Heat in general and in any internal organ (much used in the Liver Fire syndromes associated with hypertension).

- Cools the Blood (skin diseases caused by Blood Heat: hives, psoriasis, eczema, etc.).

- Dissolves Dampness, especially Damp-Heat (rash, acne, digestive system syndromes, cystitis, urethritis, fever, feeling of heaviness, loose stools, bloating, etc.).

- Swelling of the thyroid (accumulation of phlegm).

- Benefits tendons and joints (especially in the arms and shoulders).

LI 12   ZHOU LIAO – ELBOW BONE-HOLE

- Very effective for 'tennis elbow'.

LI 13   SHOU WU LI – (ARM) FIVE LI

- Sedates Liver Yang.

- Expels Dampness.

LI 14   BI NAO – UPPER ARM

- Removes obstructions from the meridian caused by Wind, Cold and Damp (Painful Obstruction Syndrome of arm and shoulder).

- Benefits the eyes (clearer and better vision).

- Dissolves Phlegm and lumps (swelling of the thyroid).

LI 15   JIAN YU – SHOULDER BONE

(Hui) Meeting point of LI channel and Yang Springing Vessel (Yang Qiao Mai)

- Beneficial effect on tendons.

- Stimulates the circulation of Qi in the meridians.

- Calms pain.

- Expels Wind.

- Main point for treating Painful Obstruction Syndrome in the shoulder, for Atrophic syndrome and paralysis of the arm.

LI 16   JU GU - GREAT BONE

(Hui) Meeting point of Yang Springing Vessel (Yang Qiao Mai)

- Helps circulate Blood around the point area.

- Removes obstructions from the meridian.

- Sedates the ascent of Rebel Qi.

- Stimulates the descent of Lung Qi

- Benefits the joints.

- Opens the chest.

LI 17   TIAN DING – CELESTIAL TRIPOD

- Effective for disturbances in the larynx and pharynx.

LI 18   FU TU – PROTUBERANCE ASSISTANT

- Benefits the throat (often used for tonsillitis, laryngitis, vocal chord polyps, aphasia, mumps, hoarse voice, swelling of the thyroid, etc.).

- Calms a cough.

- Dissolves Phlegm and lumps.

LI 19   HE JIAO – GRAIN BONE-HOLE

- Removes obstructions in the meridian.

- Expels Wind.

LI 20   YING XIANG - WELCOME FRAGRANCE

(Hui) Meeting point with LI and Stomach channel

- Local Point for all problems relating to the nose (sneezing, loss of sense of smell, nosebleeds, sinusitis, rhinorrhoea, nasal congestion, allergic rhinitis, nasal polyps, etc.).

- Expels external Wind, Cold and Heat (used in facial paralysis, trigeminal neuralgia and tic).

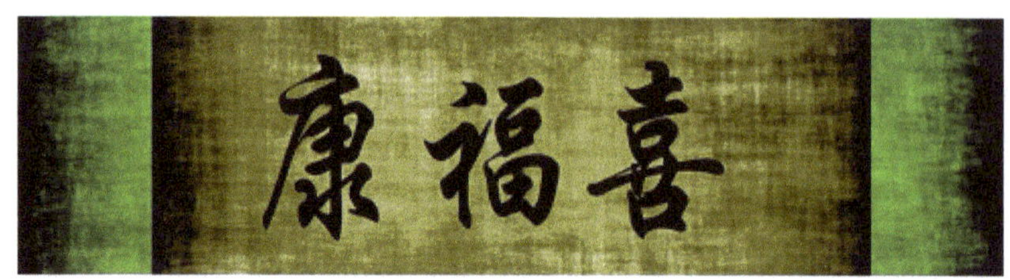

STOMACH

DIGESTION – NOURISHMENT

SHU POINT= BL21   MU POINT= CV12

07:00 to 9:00 a.m.

DIGESTIVE TRACT
REPRODUCTIVE SYSTEM
MOUTH
CHEW
APPETITE, HUNGER, DESIRE
GREED
NUTRITION
SATISFACTION
BREASTFEEDING
NURTURE
ADDICTION
DEPENDENCE
ATTACHMENT
OBSESSION, CONSTRICTION
STUBBORNNESS
WORRY
SYMPATHY
COMPASSION
RECEPTION
ACCEPTANCE
CAPACITY TO RECEIVE AND GIVE LOVE, SUPPORT AND APPRECIATE
INITIATIVE

"The Minister of the Mill", also known as The Sea of Nourishment.

FUNCTIONS

- Transforms food and fluids through a process of fermentation, sends the pure part to the Spleen and the impure part to the Small Intestine.

- Regulates, together with the Spleen, the transportation and distribution of food Qi (Stomach Yang).

- The origin of Fluids (function linked to Kidneys).

- Likes dampness and abhors dryness.

- Regulates the descent of Qi.

- Governs appetite, lactation and certain aspects of ovarian functions.

- Linked to female hormones (nutrition and menstrual cycle).

- Closely connected to Spleen.

If the Stomach is weak, so are the other organs.
Tonifying SP and ST is crucial in all cases of chronic disease and convalescence.

DISORDERS / DYSFUNCTIONS

- Sluggish digestion with stagnation of food, feeling of fullness in the epigastric area, swelling in the lower abdomen, hiccups, nausea and vomiting (counter flow of Stomach Qi - Rebel Qi).

- Stomach Fire (bad breath, sore and bleeding gums, thirst, irritability, physical and mental hyperactivity, constipation, excessive appetite, insomnia, etc.).

- Thirst, dry tongue with cracks, poor digestion (lack of liquid).

- Pain in the stomach, hyperacidity, constipation, and dry stools (Empty Heat = weak Stomach Yin).

- Problems with the mouth: ulcers and cold sores (Stomach Heat).

- Eating too much or too quickly.

- Prolonged colds, rhinitis and cough.

- Nasal congestion and sneezing.

- Eye strain from too much reading.

- Tension in the jaw, neck and shoulder area.

- Breast problems

- Irregular menstrual cycle and improper functioning of the female organs.

- Pain in the solar plexus and abdominal region.

- Tension and pain in the middle-lower back and weak abdominal muscles.

- Heavy legs and cold from the knees down.

- Easily fatigued, tired, especially in the morning.

- Yawning often.

- Latent dissatisfaction.

- Worry about the smallest details.

- Mental imbalance, delirium, confusion or hallucinations (Phlegm-Fire in the Stomach, where Fire disturbs the Shen).

- Breastfeeding difficulties.

- Poor or excessive appetite.

- Emotional attachment, addictive habits, under the influence of an addiction.

QI DEFICIENCY

Loss of appetite, epigastric discomfort, fatigue, weakness of the limbs, loose stools, etc.

Causes:
Food with insufficient or no nourishment; chronic disease; Spleen Qi Deficiency.

YIN DEFICIENCY

Lack of appetite, nausea, belching, hiccups, dry mouth and throat, feeling of fullness after meals, flushing, constipation, anxiety, difficulty in sleeping, etc.

Causes:
Irregular diet; terminal stage of febrile illness.

FIRE

Burning and epigastric pain, thirst for cold drinks, constant hunger, bulimic attacks, weight loss despite regular intake of food, digestion accelerated, inflamed gums, mouth ulcers, regurgitation, halitosis, nausea, caries, stomatitis, constipation, etc.

Causes:
Excessive consumption of hot and fatty food; emotional problems.

COLD

Cold and painful epigastric area, vomiting of clear liquids, absence of thirst, abdominal rumbling.

Causes:
Exposure to Cold; constitutional Yang Deficiency; excessive consumption of cold foods.

REBEL QI

Nausea, vomiting, hiccups, belching, etc.

Causes:
Emotional problems (anxiety, worry, brooding, etc.)

RETENTION OF FOOD

Epigastric pain and bloating, lack of appetite, nausea, vomiting, acid regurgitation, belching, bad breath, constipation or diarrhoea with undigested food, sleeplessness, etc.

Causes:
Eating in a hurry and excessive amounts of food; worry.

BLOOD STAGNATION

Stabbing epigastric pain after taking food, vomiting with blood, bloody stools, loss of appetite, etc.

Causes:
Long term emotional problems (anger, frustration, resentment, worry, depression, etc.); Stomach Fire; retention of food in the stomach, stagnation of Liver Qi; other Stomach syndromes.

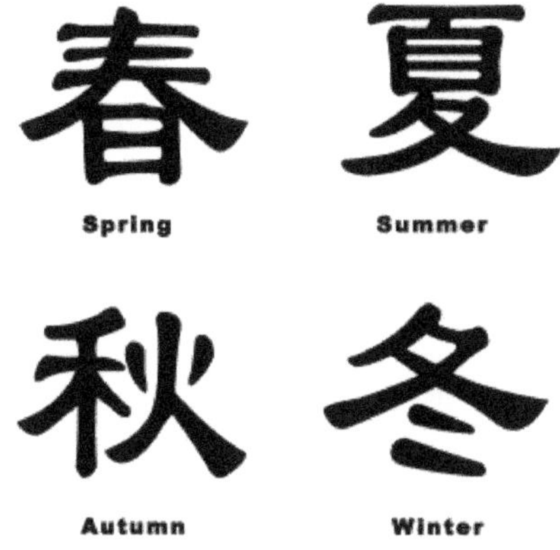

STOMACH MERIDIAN POINTS

ST 1   CHENG QI – TEAR CONTAINER

(Hui) Meeting point of the Stomach channel with the Yang Springing Vessel (Yang Qiao Mai) and Conception Vessel (Ren Mai)

For all sorts of visual disorders:

- Acute and chronic conjunctivitis, myopia, astigmatism, strabismus, night blindness and colour blindness, glaucoma, optic nerve atrophy, cataracts, keratitis and retinitis, etc.

- Stops lacrimation.

- Expels external Wind (swelling, pain, lacrimation and eyelid paralysis) and internal Wind (tic of the eyelid).

ST 2   SI BAI - FOUR WHITES

Yang Qiao Mai point

- For eye problems (as in ST1).

- Trigeminal neuralgia.

ST 3   JU LIAO – GREAT BONE HOLE

Yang Qiao Mai point

- Expels external and internal Wind (as in ST1 and ST2).

- Trigeminal neuralgia and facial paralysis.

- Action also extends to the nose (epistaxis and nasal obstruction).

- Removes obstructions from the meridian.

ST 4   DI CANG – EARTH GRANARY

Yang Qiao Mai point.
(Hui) Meeting point of Stomach and Large Intestine

- Expels external Wind (recommended for facial paralysis with deviation of the mouth).

- Removes obstructions from the meridian.

- Action on the tendons and muscles of the face (recommended for aphasia).

ST 5   DA YING - GREAT RECEPTION

-   Removes obstructions from the meridian.

-   Raises defensive Wei Qi.

-   Expels Wind.

ST 6   JI ACHE – CHEEK CARRIAGE

-   Eliminates external Wind.

-   Activates the channel.

-   Paired with SI4 - effective for facial paralysis, mumps, jaw and masseter problems, toothaches.

ST 7   XIA GUAN – BELOW THE JOINT
(Hui) Meeting point of Stomach and the Gall Bladder channels

-   Activates the meridian.

-   Effective for ear problems (otitis, deafness, ear pain).

-   Paired with ST44 - for jaw problems and toothache.

ST 8   TOU WEI – HEAD CORNER
Yang Wei Mai point
(Hui) Meeting point of Gall Bladder and Stomach channels

-   Eliminates Wind.

-   Eliminates Dampness from the head alleviating pain (frontal headaches, splitting headaches, heaviness in the head due to Dampness or Phlegm).

-   Benefits the eyes.

-   Expels Heat.

-   Stops lacrimation.

-   Relieves dizziness (caused by stagnation of Dampness or Phlegm).

ST 9   REN YING – MAN'S PROGNOSIS

(He) Sea of Qi point

-   Subdues rebellious Stomach Qi (nausea, hiccups, belching, asthma, etc.).

-   Removes obstructions from the head and stimulates the descent of Qi (Excess Syndrome in the upper part of the body).

-   Benefits the throat, removing lumps, swelling and Heat (swollen, red or sore throat, tonsillitis, pharyngitis, enlarged thyroid, etc.).

ST 10   SHUI TU - WATER PROMINENCE

-   Drains Phlegm-Heat and Dampness.

ST 11   QI SHE – QI ABODE

-   Stimulates the flow of Qi

-   Eliminates Wind and Cold.

ST 12   QUE PEN – EMPTY BASIN

-   Subdues rebellious Stomach Qi.

-   Calms the Shen (nervousness, anxiety, insomnia due to disharmony of the Stomach).

ST 13   QI HU – QI DOOR

-   Eliminates Wind.

-   Lowers rebellious Qi (dry cough, hiccups, shortness of breath, etc.).

ST 14   KU FANG - STORE ROOM

-   Drains Damp-Heat from the Middle Burner (cough with yellow sputum, chest tightness).

ST 15   WU YI – ROOF

-   Expels Heat and Humidity and Spleen Excess syndromes.

ST 16   YING CHUANG – BREAST WINDOW

-   Dispels Dampness and Heat from the centre of the body.

ST 17   RU ZHONG – BREAST CENTRE

-   Expels Wind-Damp and clears Heat

    Because of its location (centre of nipple), it is treated with delicacy and when
    appropriate.

ST 18   RU GEN – BREAST ROOT

-   Regulates Stomach Qi especially in relation to the breast (mastitis, premenstrual
    swelling, nodules, breastfeeding, etc.).

-   Eliminates stagnation.

ST 19   BU RONG – NOT CONTAINED

-   Transforms Damp obstruction in the Spleen.

-   Clears Heat that is consuming the Ying Qi (Nourishing Energy).

-   Cools the Blood.

ST 20   CHENG MAN – ASSUMING FULLNESS

-   Harmonizes the Liver and the Spleen.

-   Drains Damp-Heat in the Middle Burner.

ST 21   LIANG MEN – BEAM GATE

- Subdues rebellious Qi (Stomach Excess syndromes)

- Alleviates vomiting.

- Alleviates pain and burning in the epigastrium (paired with ST44 and ST34).

ST 22   GUAN MEN – PASS GATE

- Drains Dampness allowing the Spleen Qi to flow freely (lumps in the abdomen, pain or colic, bloating, flatulence, diarrhoea, etc).

ST 23   TAI YI - SUPREME UNITY

- Promotes the descent of Yang.

- Sedates the Shen (restlessness, madness, agitation, neurosis, etc.).

ST 24   HUAROU MEN – SLIPPERY FLESH GATE

- Promotes the descent of Yang.

- Calms the Shen.

ST 25   TIAN SHU – CELESTIAL PIVOT

Front Collection point of Large Intestine (Mu point)

- Restores the function of the intestines (stops diarrhoea and pain, constipation and heartburn).

- Mu point for acute Stomach syndromes.

- Clears Heat.

- Harmonizes the flow of Qi in the Large Intestine.

- Effective for anxiety, schizophrenia, mental excitement, madness, etc.

ST 26   WAI LING – OUTER MOUND

-   Alleviates pain and eliminates Cold invasion in the Lower Burner (severe abdominal pain, nausea, painful menstruation, etc.).

ST 27   DA JU – GREAT GIGANTIC

-   Moves Stomach Qi (in the case of Stomach Excess, Qi Stagnation in the Lower Burner).

-   For hernia and male genital problems.

ST 28   SHUI DAO – WATERWAY

-   Regulates the Qi in the Lower Burner (menstrual cycle disorders caused by Qi and Blood stasis).

-   Opens Water passages in the Lower Burner, stimulating the expulsion of fluids (difficulty in passing urine, urine retention, oedema, etc.).

ST 29   GUI LAI – RETURN

-   Eliminates Blood stasis (especially of the uterus, regulates menstruation, can start menstruation - for dysmenorrhea with blood clots, etc.).

ST 30   QI CHONG - QI THOROUGHFARE

Meeting point of Stomach and Thoroughfare Vessel (Chong Mai)
Sea of Food (Sea of Water and Grain) point

-   Regulates the Qi and Blood in the Middle Burner, the Lower Burner and genitals (pain, abdominal masses, hernias, swelling, impotence, testicular atrophy and all problems related to the uterus and genitals).

-   Harmonises Yin-Yang metabolisms (paired with KD11).

-   Stimulates Jing (as it is linked to Pre-Heaven through the Chong Mai and to the Post-Heaven).

-   Promotes the functions of digestion and food processing related to Stomach and Spleen.

ST 31   BI GUAN – THIGH JOINT

- Removes obstructions in the meridian.

- For problems of the legs (weakness, feeling cold, tingling, tension, difficulty lifting or bending the leg).

- Benefits the Kidney and expels Cold.

ST 32   FU TU – CROUCHING RABBIT

- Removes obstructions from the meridian.

- Disperses Wind-Heat in the Blood (skin diseases such as acute urticaria).

- Tonifies and activates the Liver Qi.

ST 33   YIN SHI – YIN MARKET

- Dispels Cold in the Lower Burner.

ST 34   LIANG QIU – BEAM HILL

(Xi) Cleft point of the Stomach channel

- Constrains the rebellious Stomach Qi (hiccups, nausea, vomiting, belching, etc.).

- Being a Xi point, it is recommended for painful syndromes, both acute and Excess syndromes.

- Removes obstructions from the meridian.

- Dispels Damp and the Wind from the knee joint.

ST 35   DU BI – CALF'S NOSE

- Strengthens the meridian.

- Alleviates pain.

- Reduces swelling.

- Removes Dampness and Cold.

Effective in the treatment of Painful Obstruction Syndrome of the knee.

ST 36   ZU SAN LI – LEG THREE LI

(He) Sea Point, corresponding to the Earth phase.
Sea of Food point

- Harmonizes Stomach and Spleen (tonifies the Pre-Heaven Qi).

- Tonifies the Qi and Blood in Deficiency syndromes.

- Strengthens the body (if a person is extremely weak after a chronic illnesses or long convalescence), increases resistance to external pathogenic factors.

   A preventive measure: Moxa every 5-7 days for 10 min. (Strengthens the ability to resist disease - but not recommended for those under 30 years old).

- Benefits the eyes (blurred vision or loss of vision, especially in the elderly).

- Eliminates oedema.

- Regulates the intestines (especially effective for constipation).

- Expels Cold, Wind and Damp.

- Sustains the Yang.

- For Painful Obstruction Syndrome of the knee and wrist.

ST 37   SHANG JU XU – UPPER GREAT HOLLOW

Sea of Blood point
Lower Uniting point of the Large Intestine

- Regulates LI (chronic diarrhoea, Damp-Heat syndromes of LI with foul smelling, unformed faeces, with mucus and blood).

- Calms asthma and dyspnoea (opens the chest).

ST 38   TIAO KOU - RIBBON OPENING

- Removes obstructions from the meridian.

- Dispels Wind-Damp (pain and stiffness in shoulder, knee and hip joints).

ST 39   XIA JU XU – LOWER GREAT HOLLOW

Sea of Blood point
Lower Uniting point of Small Intestine

- Regulates Stomach and Small Intestine functions (lower abdominal pain, rumbling or gurgling of the bowels, borborygmi, flatulence, murky, dark urine, diarrhoea, etc.).

- Eliminates Damp-Heat and Wind-Damp.

- Alleviates pain.

- Tonifies the Blood (along with BL11 and ST37), strengthens defensive Wei Qi and Kidney Qi.

ST 40   FENG LONG – BEAUTIFUL BULGE

Luo Connecting point of the Stomach with Spleen channel

- Transforms visible Phlegm (sputum, small subcutaneous masses, thyroid and uterine masses, etc.) and invisible Phlegm (that clouds the Shen causing mental disorders, dizziness, numbness, restlessness, etc.).

- Calm asthma, since it opens the chest and regulates breathing.

- Calm and purifies the Shen (anxiety, fear and phobia).

- Clears Heat from the Stomach (tightness, burning or knot in the stomach).

ST 41   JIE XI – RAVINE DIVIDE

(Jing) River point, corresponding to the Fire phase.
Tonification point

- Removes obstructions from the meridian such as Cold and Damp (for Painful Obstruction Syndrome of the foot).

- Being a River point, it acts on the joints (ankle problems).

- Clears Heat from the Stomach.

- Purifies Shen (draws Heat down, away from the head).

ST 42   CHONG YANG - SURGING YANG

(Yuan) Source point of the Stomach channel

- Regulates the Stomach and Spleen.

- Together with TB4 it tonifies the Middle Burner and removes the Cold from the joints.

- Calms the Shen (neurosis, mental illness, etc.).

ST 43   XIAN GU – SUNKEN VALLEY

(Shu) Stream point, corresponding to the Wood phase.

- Dispels Wind and Heat from the joints.
- Removes obstructions from the meridian.

ST 44   NEI TING – INNER COURT

(Ying) Spring point, corresponding to the Water phase.

- Clears Heat from the Stomach (bleeding gums and any problem caused by Heat).
- Alleviates the feeling of fullness.
- Regulates Qi.
- Alleviates pain along the meridian (particularly in the jaw).
- Aids digestion.
- Dispels Wind from the face (facial paralysis, trigeminal neuralgia), along with SI4.

ST 45   LI DUI – SEVERE MOUTH

(Jing) Well point, corresponding to the Metal phase
Dispersion point

- Calms the Shen and Stomach (very effective for insomnia)
- Benefits the eyes
- Purifies the Heart
- Eliminates food retention

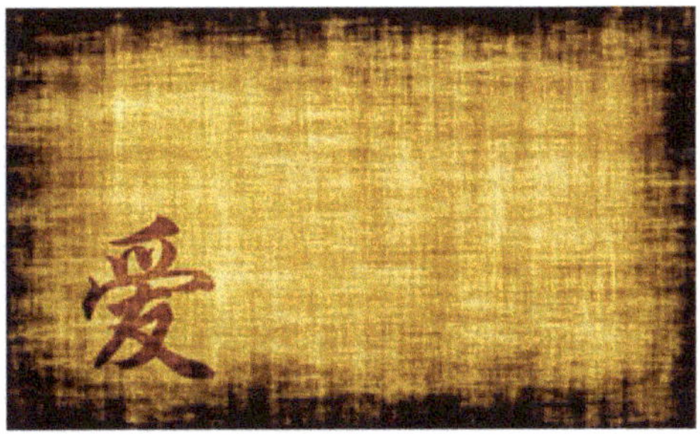

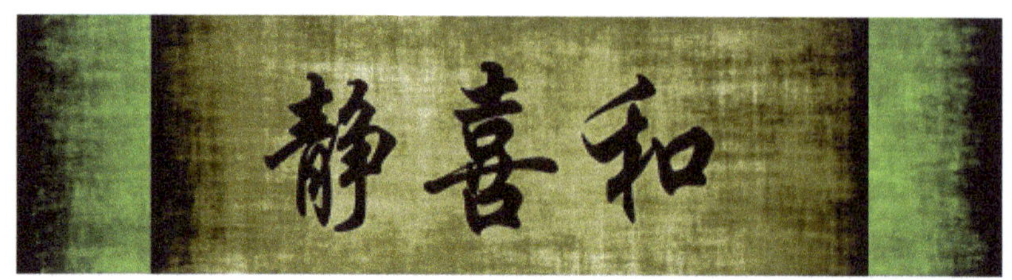

SPLEEN

TRANSFORMATION

SHU POINT = BL20   **MU POINT= LV13**

09:00 to 11:00 a.m.

FORM
STRUCTURE
STRENGTH
SUPPORT
CENTRALITY
NUTRITION
ASSIMILATION
STAGES
CYCLES
MEETING POINT BETWEEN HIGH AND LOW (FIRE-WATER)
CAPACITY TO RECEIVE AND GIVE LOVE AND SUPPORT
CONCERN
BROODING
ANALYSE
JUDGEMENT
DIGEST
CRAVES SWEET FOODS

The Minister of the granary.

The officer in charge of distribution, the carrier of energy.

<u>**FUNCTIONS**</u>

- Transformation of food in Qi (Gu Qi) and Blood (in the Heart).

- Processing, separation and diffusion of liquids.

- Distribution to the various organs and viscera.

- Regulates Blood.

- Ensures the firmness of the blood vessels (Spleen Qi ensures that blood remains in the vessels) and of the flesh, the physical form (mass and muscle tone).

- Provides for the thermal regulation of the body, through the dissemination of the Blood.

- Spleen regulates the ascent of Qi.

- Governs the centre, cycles, the steps, the changes.

- Seat of the Yi (intellect, purpose or thought): ability to organize and structure a thought, give shape and solidity, structure; to make ideas become reality; ability to concentration.

- Opens in the mouth and is manifested in the lips: moist, pink, fleshy (Deficit: thin and dry; Blood deficiency: very pale; Blood stasis: purple).

- Linked to the reproductive system (hormones, mammary glands and ovaries).

- Responsible for analytical thinking, concentration, cognition.

- Nurturing qualities: to receive and give love and support.

<u>**DISORDERS / DYSFUNCTIONS**</u>

- Digestive disorders, burping.

- Poor appetite (Qi deficiency, insufficient to transform the food).

- Feeling tired or sleepy after meals.

- Intestinal irregularities (diarrhoea: Qi deficiency, insufficient to complete digestion; constipation: lack of liquids).

- Bloating, colitis, irritable bowel syndrome.

- Bloating and abdominal pain (Qi deficiency, insufficient to move food).

- Oedema (in the lower part of the body - Yang deficiency).

- Gastric or duodenal ulcers, gastritis, enteritis, hepatitis, dysentery or nephritis.

- Overweight or too thin.

- General weakness, fatigue, lethargy.

- Muscular atrophy.

- Disorders related to blood: anaemia, bleeding (nasal, uterine, blood in stool, etc.), menstruation, etc.

- Varicose veins.

- Haemorrhoids.

- Prolapse of all organs.

- Difficulty passing urine (Yang deficiency).

- White vaginal discharge (Yang deficiency).

- Cold limbs, particularly hands and feet (Yang deficiency).

- Pain in the back and knees (difficulty standing or sitting).

- Shoulder articulation disorders ('frozen shoulder').

- Tongue: swollen, moist and pale (Yang deficiency).

- Dry, pasty mouth, pale tongue with thin white coating (Yang deficiency).

- Overthinking, ruminating.

- Inability to nurture affection, or take care of others.

Spleen must always be treated when the disease or disorder relates to Body Fluids.

If a person has had their Spleen removed the Spleen Meridian will tend to over work in order to make up for the lack of the organ.

Spleen and Stomach are closely linked. Often Stomach points are used to tonify the Spleen.

QI DEFICIENCY

Nausea, lack of appetite, bloating after meals, feeling of heaviness, loose stools, diarrhoea, fatigue, limb weakness, swelling and oedema/oedema, lethargy, pale and yellowish complexion, etc.

Causes:

Constitutional predisposition; unbalanced diet (excessive consumption of cold foods, irregular meals, the quantity and quality of food, etc.); climate with low humidity; excessive exercise; excessive mental activity (brooding, ruminating, worrying, etc.); chronic diseases, which weaken the Spleen and consequently create the formation of Phlegm.

EMPTY YANG

Same symptoms of Qi Deficiency, but more aggravated, and with symptoms of Cold.

Causes:
Chronic Spleen Qi Deficiency; prolonged exposure to Cold-Damp.

COLLAPSE OF QI

All the symptoms of the Qi Deficiency, also, dizziness, shortness of breath, asthma, weak voice, abnormal heartbeat, spontaneous sweating, visual blurring, prolapse of the abdominal organs (Stomach, uterus, anus, vagina), hernias, incontinence, etc.

Causes:
The same as for Qi Deficiency; chronic diarrhoea, prolonged stress; standing for long periods.

SPLEEN FAILS TO RETAIN THE BLOOD

Same symptoms as for Qi Deficiency, but also subcutaneous bleeding, blood in the urine and/or faeces, menorrhagia or metrorrhagia (menstrual spotting), bleeding haemorrhoids, etc.

Causes:
The same as Qi or Yang Deficiency.

DAMP-COLD

Loss of appetite, bloating and abdominal pain, nausea and vomiting, diarrhoea, lack of thirst, urinary retention, white vaginal discharge, tiredness, heaviness in the head, feeling cold epigastrium, etc.

Causes:
Prolonged exposure to Cold and Damp; incorrect diet (excessive consumption of raw and cold foods).

DAMP-HEAT

Loss of appetite, feeling of heaviness, nausea and vomiting, thirst without desire to drink, abdominal pain, flatulence, loose stools and / or the presence of blood, scanty, dark urine, mild fever, constant pain and / or anal burning, headache, etc.

Causes:
Prolonged exposure to Damp and Heat; incorrect diet (excessive consumption of alcohol, sugar and fat).

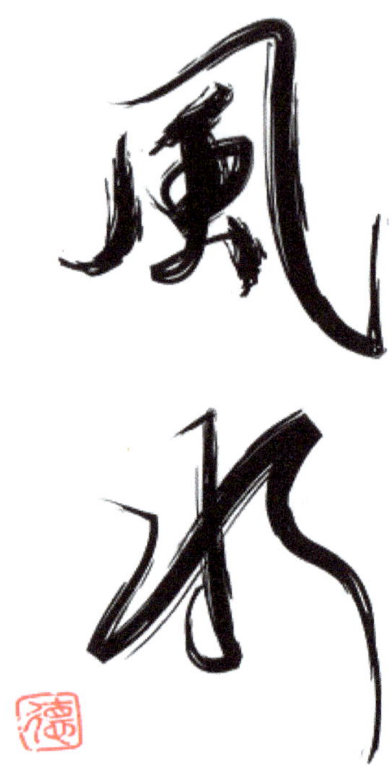

SPLEEN MERIDIAN POINTS

SP 1   YIN BAI – HIDDEN WHITE

(Jing) Well point, corresponding to the Wood phase.

- Fortifies the Spleen and Stomach.
- Regulates the Blood (especially in cases of Blood Stasis in the uterus).
- Calms Shen and dream disturbed sleep.
- For bleeding anywhere in the body, especially in the uterus (use Moxa).
- Depression and mental restlessness.

SP 2   DA DU – GREAT METROPOLIS

(Ying) Spring point, corresponding to Fire phase
Tonification point

- Fortifies the Spleen.

- Facilitates digestion.

- Clears Heat (promotes sweating in the case of fever).

SP 3   TAI BAI -   SUPREME WHITE

(Shu) Stream point
(Yuan) Source point, corresponding to the Earth phase.

- Effective in tonification of the Spleen (Deficit syndromes) because it is the Source point of the meridian and the Earth point of an Earth meridian.

- It stimulates intellectual abilities related to Spleen and is very suitable in cases of excessive mental activity, which has weakened the Spleen Qi.

- Drains Damp in the Upper Burner (confused mind, choking sensation in the chest), the Middle Burner (feeling of fullness in the epigastrium, lack of appetite) and Lower Burner (difficulty passing cloudy urine, vaginal discharge).

- Treats chronic retention of Phlegm in the Lungs (strengthening Earth to nourish Metal).

- Treats chronic pain of the spine.

SP 4   GONG SUN – YELLOW EMPEROR

Luo point
Intersection point with Thoroughfare Vessel (Chong Mai)

- Tonifies the Stomach and Spleen.

- Regulates and activates Chong Mai (Sea of Blood).

- Alleviates bleeding (because it reinforces the functions of the Spleen to contain Blood).

- Eliminates the feeling of fullness in the abdomen (and for Excess syndromes).

- Removes obstructions.

- Regulates the menstrual cycle.

- Treats urogenital problems.

SP 5   SHANG QIU - SHANG HILL (METAL)

(Jing) River point, corresponding to the Metal phase
Dispersion point

- Strengthens the Stomach and Spleen.

- Drains dampness.

- Very effective for the Painful Obstruction Syndrome caused by Dampness in any
  meridian, especially knee and ankle.

SP 6   SAN YIN JIAO -   THREE YIN INTERSECTION

(Hui) Meeting point with Kidney and Liver channels
Luo connecting point of the three Yin meridians of the foot

<u>DO NOT TREAT in first three months of pregnancy.</u>

- Strengthens the Spleen (in Deficit syndromes: lack of appetite, fatigue, loose stools,
  etc.).

- Drains Dampness (from both Cold and Heat), especially in Lower Burner (vaginal
  discharge, itching, mucus in the stools, or difficulty passing cloudy urine, etc.).

- Stimulates the functions of the liver and the free flow of Liver Qi, especially in the case
  of stagnation.

- Tonifies the kidneys, especially the Kidney Yin (vertigo, tinnitus, night sweats, feeling
  hot, dry mouth, etc.).

- Nourishes the Blood and Yin.

- Resolves Phlegm blockages.

- Aids urination (pain, difficulty, retention).

- Regulates the uterus and menstrual cycle.

- Activates the circulation of Blood and eliminates stagnation, especially in the Lower
  Burner (blood clots in menstrual blood, blood in stools, etc.).

- Cools the Blood in cases of external and internal Heat (some skin diseases).

- Alleviates pain and removes blockages, especially in the lower abdomen (this point is
  very effective).

- Calms Shen, calms irritability (obsessive thoughts, insomnia).

- For any gynaecological disturbances (regulates the uterus and the menstrual cycle),
  alleviates pain and drains Dampness (leucorrhoea (vaginal haemorrhage), menorrhagia
  and dysmenorrhea).

- Combined with ST36, it vigorously strengthens the Qi of the Middle Burner and
  particularly the Qi and Blood, helps with chronic fatigue.

- Relaxes the perineum and the pelvic floor (helps during labour).

- Stimulates the descent of Qi.

SP 7   LOU GU -   LEAKING VALLEY

- Removes Phlegm from the Lungs.

- Stimulates the circulation of Spleen and Stomach.

SP 8   DI JI – EARTH'S CRUX

(Xi) Cleft point

- Removes obstructions from the meridian (as do all Xi points).

- Regulates the Qi and Blood.

- Regulates the uterus (effective for chronic dysmenorrhea).

- Relieves pain.

SP 9   YIN LING QUAN - YIN MOUND SPRING

(He) Uniting point, corresponding to the Water phase

- Expels Damp in the Lower Burner (both Cold and Heat).

- Benefits the Lower Burner (vaginal discharge, diarrhoea, oedema in the abdomen or legs, difficulty in urination, retention, pain, cloudy urine).

- Removes obstructions from the meridian.

- Used in the Painful Obstruction Syndrome of the knee, especially if due to Dampness (swollen knee).

- Linked to menstruation: scanty menstruation, stimulates the arrival, premenstrual syndrome (headaches, irritability, bad mood, etc.).

- Helps eliminate kidney stones (combined with BL28 and BL23).

SP 10   XUE HAI -   SEA OF BLOOD

- Cools the Blood (for Heat syndromes that cause skin diseases such as eczema, hives, rashes, etc.).

- Removes Blood stasis, especially in the uterus (dysmenorrhea acute or chronic).

- Regulates the menstrual cycle.

- Invigorates the Blood (strengthens the function of the spleen to control the blood and to keep it within the blood vessels).

For knee complaints.

Poor circulation (Stagnation of Blood = Stagnation of Qi).

Easy bruising, hematoma.

SP 11   JI MEN – WINNOWER GATE

-   Benefits the bladder (micturition disorders, urinary retention, enuresis, etc.).

SP 12   CHONG MEN – SURGING GATE

(Hui) Meeting point with the Spleen and Liver channels and the Yin Linking Vessel (Yin Wei Mai).

-   Removes obstructions of the meridian.

-   Nourishes the Yin.

-   Useful in the treatment of the Painful Obstruction Syndrome of the flank (pain that extends to the groin).

-   Moves Qi in the abdomen, especially in the case of Cold.

-   Combined with ST30 harmonizes the arterio-venous flow.

-   For Blood poisoning (poisons, etc.).

-   Invigorates Bladder and Kidney Qi.

SP 13   FU SHE – BOWEL ABODE

(Hui) Meeting point of the Spleen and Liver channels with the Yin Linking Vessel (Yin Wei Mai)

-   Regulates fluid metabolism (retention, lumps and masses in the abdomen, oedema, etc.).

-   Invigorates Spleen and Bladder.

SP14   FU JIE – ABDOMINAL BIND

-   Drains Damp-Cold.

SP 15   DA HENG – GREAT HORIZONTAL

(Hui) Meeting point with the Yin Linking Vessel (Yin Wei Mai)

- Strengthens the Spleen in its functions of processing and dissemination.

- Fortifies the limbs (cold, weak limbs).

- Dissolves Damp (chronic diarrhoea with mucus in the stool).

- Regulates the Qi in the abdomen and promotes the flow of Liver Qi.

- Relieves abdominal pain.

- Stimulates the function of the Large Intestine (chronic constipation).

Important for abdominal disorders.

SP 16   FU AI – ABDOMINAL LAMENT

(Hui) Meeting point with the Yin Linking Vessel (Yin Wei Mai)

- Relieves Cold depletion of the Spleen (severe pain in the abdomen, constipation, diarrhoea, etc.).

SP 17   SHI DOU – FOOD HOLE

- Drains massive accumulations of Dampness.

SP18   TIAN XI – CELESTIAL RAVINE

- Tonifies the Spleen Qi.

SP 19   XIONG XIANG – CHEST VILLAGE

- Relieves pain and tension in the chest.

SP 20   ZHON YING – ALL-ROUND FLOURISHING

- Drains Damp-Heat from Lungs.

SP 21   DA BAO – GREAT EMBRACEMENT

Great Luo point of the Spleen

- Intensifies the contact between the primary Spleen channel and the Luo channels of the Spleen.

- Mobilizes the Blood in Luo Xue.

- Works on all blockages.

In cases of Blood stasis in Luo meridians (symptoms: muscle pain that migrates from one part of the body to another).

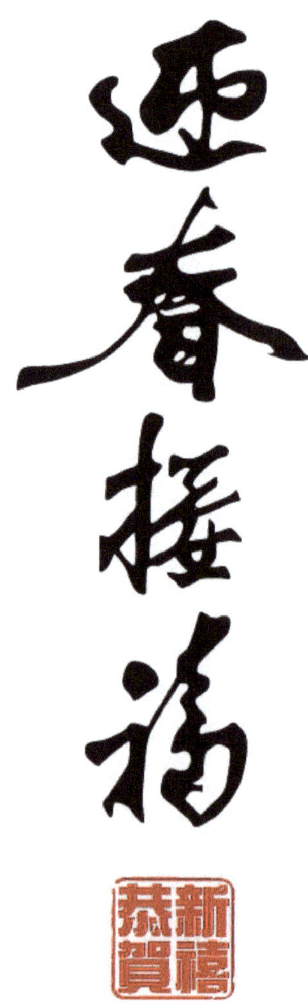

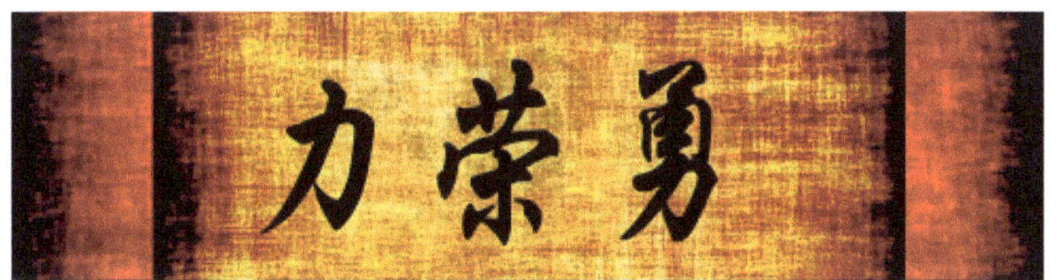

HEART

INTERPRETATION

SHU POINT = BL15   **MU POINT = CV14**

11:00 a.m. to 1:00 p.m.

AWARENESS
INTUITION
INTROSPECTION
SELF ESTEEM
DEEP INTERNAL CHANGES
TRANSITION
CAPACITY OF DISCERNMENT
WISDOM
EMOTIONS
COMPASSION
JOY
LOVE
INNER PEACE
BALANCE
HARMONY
WILL-POWER
LAUGHTER
FACE COMPLEXION

The Emperor, the sovereign ruler, excellent at introspection and interpretation, issues orders.

The supreme controller who oversees the functions of the Body-Mind-Spirit.

- Formation of Blood: it receives Gu Qi from SP and ST and turns it into Blood.
  The Fire (Yang) generates the Blood (Yin), which in turn cools the Heart, preventing
  Fire from rising.

- Circulation of Blood: as material, energetic and spiritual nourishment.
  Heart Qi gives Blood the impetus to circulate in the blood vessels.

- Regulates sweating (Blood and Body Fluids or Jin-Ye have a common origin and
  mutual exchange).

- The sensory organ associated with the Heart is the tongue (colour, shape and the tip
  indicates its condition).

  Blood Deficiency: pale, thin tongue.
  Blood Stagnation: purple tongue.
  Heat: dry, dark red tongue with ulcerations.

- The Heart is where the Shen (spirit) resides (mental faculties, awareness, consciousness)
  and how it is spread.

- The Heart is the centre of an individual's life and its guiding light. It is the link between
  the human being and heaven, the divine.

- Governs the Blood, which is the root of Shen.

- Connected to sleep and dreams (profound expression of the Shen).

- It is manifested in the face (Blood plentiful and strong Heart = rosy, radiant
  complexion).

- Associated with the eyes (they manifest the Shen).

DISORDERS / DYSFUNCTIONS

- Poor blood circulation (cold hands, pale face).

- Fire rising (agitation, restlessness, insomnia, mental disorders to delirium).

- Excessive, profuse, spontaneous sweating (Heart Qi deficiency) or night sweats (Yin or
  Heart Blood deficiency).

- Speech disorders (aphasia, stuttering, talking incessantly and unprovoked, nervous
  repeated laughter = Heart Fire).

- Cardiovascular disorders, palpitations, tachycardia.

- Anaemia.

- Hypertension.

- Hyperthyroidism.

- Memory loss.

- Insomnia, excessive dreaming, neurosis, restlessness.

- Blood deficiency (pale face and tongue, dizziness, lethargy, difficulty falling asleep). Often associated with Spleen Qi deficiency (since it produces the Blood).

- Yin deficiency (reddish tongue, night sweats, hot palms of hands and soles of the feet, agitation, frequent nocturnal wakening). Often associated with Kidney Yin deficiency (source of Yin of all organs).

- Shock, coma, amnesia, mental illnesses such as schizophrenia (dispersion or disappearance of Shen).

- Epilepsy (Phlegm in the Heart).

HEART QI DEFICIENCY

Paleness, asthenia, palpitations (during the day), difficulty breathing (dyspnoea), sweating, etc.

Causes:
Emotional problems (sadness, excessive excitement, excessive feelings, etc.); severe or prolonged bleeding; advanced age.

BLOOD DEFICIENCY

Insomnia (difficulty sleeping), dizziness, anxiety, tendency to be afraid, poor memory, palpitations (frequently in the evening), pale and dull complexion, etc.

Causes:
Excessive anxiety and worry; severe bleeding; poor nutrition (Spleen Deficit); diminished Jing and Kidney Yin in advancing age.

BLOOD STAGNATION

Chest oppression and pain that radiates to the left arm; tongue and lips purple, cold hands, etc.

Causes:
Long term repression of emotions, excess emotion; Cold invasion; catarrh; excessive fatigue.

HEART YANG DEFICIENCY

Pale face, cold extremities, palpitations, dyspnoea, shortness of breath, palpitations, fatigue, feeling of tightness in the chest, etc.

<u>Causes:</u>

The same as in Qi deficiency; as well as chronic Kidney Yang deficiency.

HEART YIN DEFICIENCY

Insomnia (difficulty falling asleep and disturbed sleep), mental restlessness, anxiety, irritability, sensation of heat in the extremities, night sweats, poor memory, palpitations, etc. (N.B in cases of Yin deficiency, there is always a Blood deficiency).

<u>Causes:</u>

Associated to or secondary to Kidney Yin deficiency; excessive anxiety and long term worry, overly active life; invasion of external Heat that consumes Body Fluids.

FIRE ATTACKING HEART

Agitation, insomnia, palpitations, restlessness, mental, verbal delirium, mouth and tongue ulcers, red face, thirst, blood in urine or dark urine, etc.

<u>Causes:</u>

Long term excess of emotions (anxiety, depression, worry, sadness, etc.) causes a stagnation of Qi, that, in the long term, it becomes Fire; Liver Fire (linked to anger, resentment, frustration, etc.); a serious deficiency affecting all the Yin.

PHLEGM

Mental disorders and mental restlessness, palpitations, verbal delirium, hysteria, insomnia, dream disturbed sleep, violent behaviour and agitated depression, etc.

<u>Causes:</u>

Long term Qi stagnation can turn into Fire, which causes the consumption of Body Fluids and the formation of Phlegm; external Heat and a diet rich of hot, spicy and fatty foods (causing Phlegm-Fire).

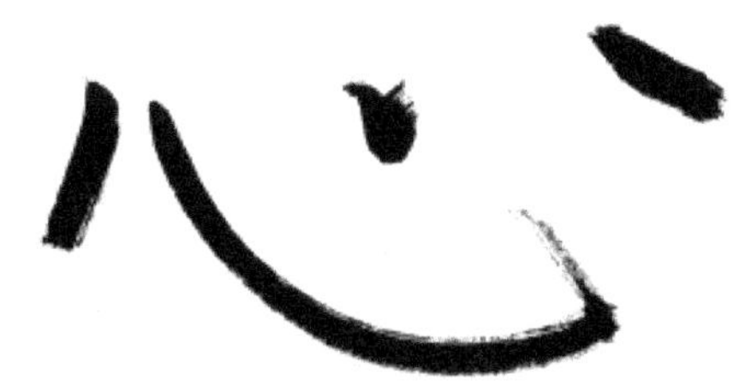

HEART MERIDIAN POINTS

HT 1   JI QUAN – HIGHEST SPRING

- Nourishes Heart Yin and clears Empty-Heat (night sweats, dry mouth, mental restlessness, insomnia, agitation, etc.).

- Used in cases of a stroke with paralysis of the arm.

HT 2   QING LING QUAN – GREEN-BLUE SPIRIT

- Tonifies the Liver Yin and activates Liver Yang.

HT 3   SHAO HAI – LESSER SEA

(He) Uniting point, corresponding to the Water phase

- Expels Heart Fire, effective in calming the Shen at a mental level (epilepsy, severe depression, mental retardation, mood swings).

- Removes obstructions from the meridian (Painful Obstruction Syndrome, Atrophic Syndrome, Cerebrovascular accident)

HT 4   LING DAO – SPIRIT PATHWAY

(Jing) River point, corresponding to the Metal phase

- Removes obstructions from the meridian.

As a River point it has a specific action on the joints and bones (spasms and pain in the forearm and elbow and wrist arthritis).

HT 5   TONG LI –CONNECTING LI

Luo point of the Heart channel

- Main point to tonify Heart Qi with a special effect on speech (aphasia).
- Benefits the Bladder: being a Luo point it provides a link with SI, which in turn connects with BL in Tai Yang (Bladder Heat: thirst, bitter mouth, insomnia, ulcers of the tongue, burning urination and presence of blood in urine).
- Calms the Shen (mild depression and sadness).
- Connected to the capacity to forgive.

HT 6   YIN XI – YIN CLEFT

(Xi) Cleft point

- Nourishes the Heart Yin (insomnia, night sweats, dry mouth, etc.).
- Reduces sweating (Empty Heart Yin). Treat in conjunction with KD7.
- Clears Heat (mental restlessness, agitation, sensation of heat in the face, etc.).
- Calms the Shen.

HT 7   SHEN MEN – SPIRIT GATE

(Shu) Stream point
(Yuan) Source point
Dispersion point
Most important point on the Heart meridian.

- Calms the Shen (for any Heart syndrome - more effective in men).
- Also affects memory and mental capacity (eg. mental retardation in children).

- Nourishes the Blood and Heart Yin (Heart Blood deficiency: anxiety, worry, insomnia, poor memory, palpitations and pale tongue).

- Clears Heat.

HT 7	**PC 7**
Both nourish the Heart Blood and calm the Shen	
More indicated for Deficit syndromes	Best for Excess syndromes
Not suitable for diseases caused by Heat	Important in cases of diseases caused by Heat
Slight action in calming the Shen	More effective for anxiety and severe mania
Does not open the orifices of the Heart	Opens the orifices of the Heart
More effective in men	More effective for women, particularly for emotional problems caused by the break-up of a relationship

---

HT8   SHAO FU – LESSER MANSION

(Ying) Spring point, corresponding to the Fire phase.

- Clears Fire, Empty-Heat and Phlegm-Fire (very effective for Full/Excess Heart syndromes: insomnia, excessive dreaming, thirst, bitter mouth, mental restlessness, mood swings, dark urine, tongue ulcers, red tongue with red tip and yellow coating).

- Calms the Shen, but only in syndromes with Excess Heart Heat (also for more serious mental problems such as schizophrenia and psychosis).

- Restores the state of consciousness.

HT 9   SHAO CHONG – LESSER SURGE

(Jing) Well point, corresponding to theWood phase.
Tonification point

- Subdues Internal Wind (Cerebro-vascular attack).

- Clears Heat (Excess Heart Heat syndromes).

- Opens the orifices of the Heart when blocked by internal Wind.

- Relieves the feeling of fullness in the area of the heart.

- Restores the state of consciousness.

- Purifies the Heart.

- Calms the Shen (severe anxiety, hysteria).

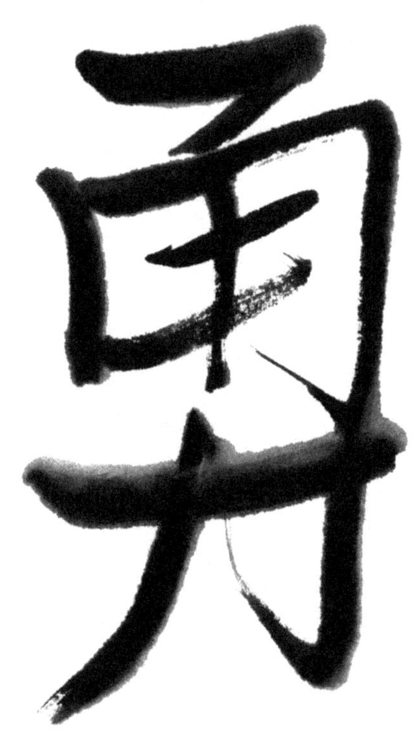

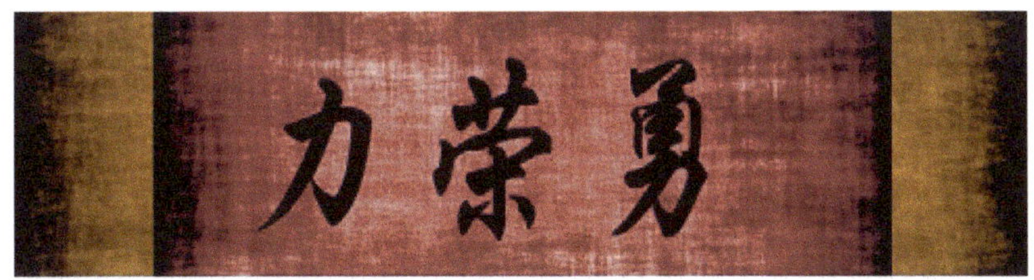

SMALL INTESTINE

ASSIMILATION

SHU POINT = BL27   **MU POINT = CV4**

1:00 to 3:00 p.m.

ABSORPTION
INTERPRETATION
CAPACITY OF DISCERNMENT
SHOCK
EMOTIONS
COMPASSION
LOVE
JOY
LAUGHTER
INTROSPECTION
RE-EVALUATION OF SELF
GREAT INTERNAL CHANGES
TRANSITIONS
STRONG DETERMINATION
WHIPLASH
PATIENCE

The root of the Heart (a branch of the Heart passes in the SI and a branch of the SI passes through the Heart).

The separator of the pure from the impure (at all levels of experience).

The Alchemist.

FUNCTIONS

- The Small Intestine receives food and liquids from the Stomach and Spleen where they have been digested, and transforms them again, separating the pure and the impure. It then sends the liquids to the Bladder, and the solids to the Large Intestine.

- Affects urinary function due to its direct functional relationship with the Bladder.

- The pure fluids from the SI nourish the Heart and blood vessels.

- Helps the Heart to keep the Qi in the Hara so as to foster calm and tranquillity.

- Correlated with the function of the ovaries and with maintaining the regularity of the menstrual cycle.

- Affects mental clarity, the capacity of good judgment and discernment in order to make correct decisions.

- Works in conjunction with the Heart to integrate sensory and emotional stimuli from the external environment into body-mind to be then further integrated into the Blood, into the flesh and into the internal responses of the individual.

DISORDERS / DYSFUNCTIONS

- Anaemia.

- Keeping things pent up inside, as in concealing anger or denying a state of shock. This causes a stagnation of energy in the neck and shoulder area, the person gets tired quickly, lower back pain and leg cramps.

- Menstrual disorders, migraines and neurotic symptoms associated with maternity or after a difficult birth.

- Thirst, bitter taste in mouth, tongue ulceration and blood in the urine (Heart Fire that is transmitted to SI).

- Urinary problems (Heart Fire transmitted to the Bladder via SI).

- Shoulder pain, tension and stiff neck.

- Frozen shoulder.

- Whiplash.

- Problems with hearing (ringing in ears, hearing loss or ear infections).

- Shock (blood flows to vital organs when there is a limb injury and causes stagnation of blood in the abdomen).

- Dissociation or disharmony between the upper and lower body (cold pelvic area and legs and hot face, or weakness in lower half of the body and heavy legs).

- Appendicitis.

- Lower back pain.

- Dysmenorrhea and gynaecological diseases.

HEAT

Urination problems (difficulty, pain, blood, etc.), scanty, dark urine, abdominal pain, discomfort and heat in the chest, sore throat, mouth ulcers, deafness, mental restlessness, etc.

Causes:
Long term emotional problems (anxiety, stress, excessive commitments, etc.).
Inappropriate diet.

COLD

Abdominal pain, borborygmi, diarrhoea, frequent urination, clear, abundant urine, desire for hot drinks, etc.

Causes:
Excessive consumption of cold and raw foods; invasion of external Cold.

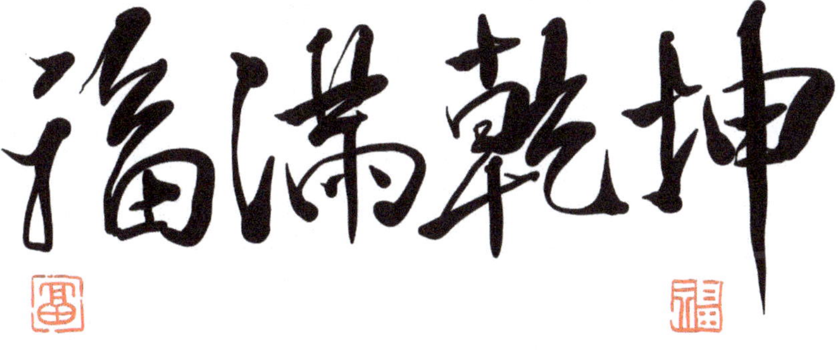

THE SMALL INTESTINE MERIDIAN POINTS

SI 1   SHAO ZE - LESSER MARSH

(Jing) Well point, corresponding to the Metal phase.

- Eliminates Wind-Heat, especially with symptoms in the head and neck (chronic stiff neck, torticollis, headache).

- Effective in acute tonsillitis from external Wind-Heat.

- Encourages the regaining of the consciousness in cases of internal Wind and Phlegm that obstruct the orifices, as in a Cerebro-Vascular attack (with loss of consciousness).

- Stimulates lactation after childbirth, especially in syndromes of Excess (the presence of pathogenic factors or Liver Qi stagnation, which inhibits the production of milk).

SI2   QIAN GU – FRONT VALLEY

(Ying) Spring point, corresponding to the Water phase.

- Expels both internal and external Heat (being a Spring point).

SI 3   HOU XI – BACK RAVINE / BACK STREAM

(Shu) Stream point, corresponding to the Wood phase.
Confluent point by means of which the Governing Vessel (Du Mai) is opened.
Tonification point.

- To treat all the symptoms relating to the Governing Vessel (Du Mai), in particular it eliminates the interior Wind from the Du Mai (tremors, convulsions, epilepsy, dizziness, headache, stiff neck, etc.).

- Eliminates exterior Wind, Heat or Cold, relaxes muscles and tendons (neck stiffness, occipital headache, back pain, fever, chills, etc.).

- Effects the muscles and tendons that are located along the meridians of Governing Vessel (Du Mai), SI and BL.

- With BL62- acts on the entire spine in both acute and chronic conditions, if the pain is on the spine or on both sides.

- Activates the Du Mai and tonifies the Kidneys (more appropriate for men rather than for women).

- Dispels Damp in the chest and in the GB that can cause jaundice and feelings of suffocation and tightness in the chest.

-   Purifies the Shen, because, through the Governing Vessel (Du Mai) it acts on the brain (it helps to strengthen decisional powers, mental clarity and good judgment).

SI 4   WAN GU – WRIST BONE

(Yuan) Source point.

-   Removes obstructions from the meridian (for Painful Obstruction Syndrome of the wrist and elbow).

-   Treats jaundice caused by Damp-Heat obstructing the GB, hypochondriac pain and inflammation of the gallbladder.

-   Clears Phlegm.

SI 5   YANG GU – YANG VALLEY

(Jing) River point, corresponding to the Fire phase.

-   Purifies the Shen, or rather helps to have mental clarity and to make choices in a specific moment in life.

-   Expels Wind-Heat.

-   Removes obstructions from the meridian (as does SI4).

-   Dispels Dampness from the knees when they are swollen and hot.

SI 6   YANG LAO – NURSING THE AGED

(Xi) Cleft point.

-   Removes obstructions from the meridian, relaxing tendons and ligaments that cause stiffness in the neck or shoulders.

-   Clears vision, but only if the syndromes are related to Heart or SI (diminished sight, visual disturbances, blurred vision).

SI 7   ZHI ZHENG – BRANCH TO THE CORRECT

Luo Connecting point of the Small Intestine.

- For any problem along this meridian (especially for severe pain in the elbow).

- Calms the Shen in cases of neurosis, fear, severe anxiety (being a Luo connecting point through a branch that links it to the Heart meridian).

SI 8   XIAO HAI -   SMALL SEA

(He) Uniting point, corresponding to the Earth phase.
Dispersion point.

- Removes obstructions from the meridian (Painful Obstruction Syndrome of the elbow and neck).

- Disperses Damp-Heat. Effective for acute swelling of glands in the neck, and for mumps.

- Calms the Shen.

SI 9   JIAN ZHEN – TRUE SHOULDER
- Local point for disorders of the shoulder (Painful Obstruction Syndrome).

SI 10   NAO SHU – UPPER ARM TRANSPORT

Meeting point of the SI channel with the Yang Springing Vessel (Yang Qiao Mai) and the Yang Linking Vessels (Yang Wei Mai)

- For Painful Obstruction Syndrome of the shoulder (it helps when joint mobility is compromised).

- Expels Wind and Damp

SI 11   TIAN ZONG – CELESTIAL GATHERING
- For Painful Obstruction Syndrome of the shoulder.

- Dispels Wind and Damp.

SI 12   BING FENG – GRASPING THE WIND

Meeting point of the meridians of SI, LI, HT, GB, TB and ST channels.

- Expels Wind (stiffness and shoulder pain).

SI 13   QU YUAN – CROOKED WALL

- Obstruction causing pain in the shoulder and neck.
- Dispels Wind and cools Heat (stiffness, pain and heat in the shoulder, pain radiating to the shoulder and/or arm).

SI 14   JIAN WAI SHU - OUTER SHOULDER TRANSPORT

- Obstruction causing pain in shoulder and neck.

SI 15   JIAN ZHONG SHU - CENTRAL SHOULDER TRANSPORT

Similar to the preceding points, but used less often.

SI 16   TIAN CHUANG – CELESTIAL WINDOW

Window of Heaven point.
- Expels Wind.
- Harmonises Liver Qi.

SI 17   TIAN RONG – CELESTIAL COUNTENANCE

Window of Heaven point.

- Drains Damp, expels external or internal Heat (indicated by swelling of the cervical glands, mumps and tonsils).

SI 18   **QUAN LIAO – CHEEK BONE-HOLE**

The Meeting point of the SI and TB meridians.

- Expels Wind, especially when it affects the face (facial paralysis, tics, trigeminal
  neuralgia, etc.).

SI 19   **TING GONG – AUDITORY PALACE**

The Meeting point of the SI, GB and TB meridians.

- Important local point for tinnitus and deafness (especially if caused by Heart or Lung
  Qi Deficiency).

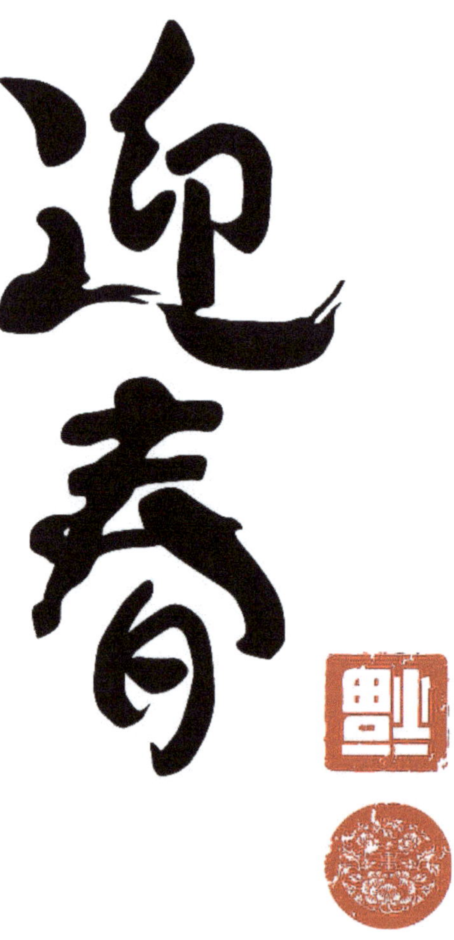

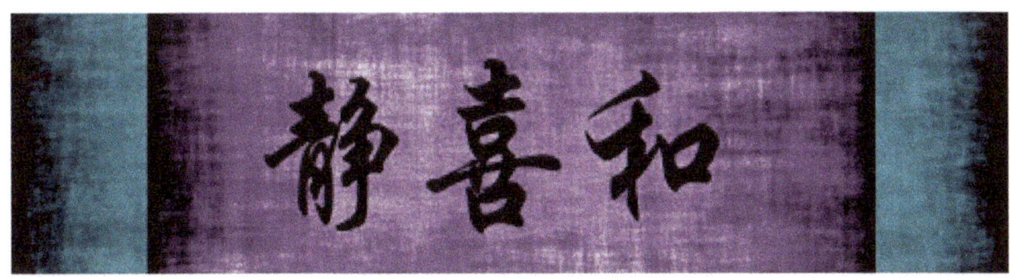

BLADDER

PURIFICATION

SHU POINT = BL 28 *   **MU POINT = CV3**

* Located 1.5 cm lateral to the 2nd sacral vertebra (not to be treated during pregnancy)

3:00 p.m. to 5:00 p.m.

AUTONOMIC NERVOUS SYSTEM
PITUITARY GLAND,
GROWTH
DRIVE, IMPETUS
FEAR
ANXIETY, TENSION
STRESS
HYPERACTIVITY
AGITATION
BREAKDOWN
NEUROSIS
PARANOIA
INSECURITY
BONES, JOINTS
TIREDNESS, FATIGUE
PURIFICATION OF FLUIDS
JEALOUSY, SUSPICION
RESENTMENT
REPRESSED SEXUAL DESIRES

District Officer in charge of collecting and eliminating waste liquids and energetic impurities (fear, emotions, negative thoughts, etc.)

FUNCTIONS

- Transforms the impure liquids it receives from SP and SI, and thanks to the Qi and Heat provided by the Kidney Yang, eliminates the urine, retaining the pure liquids.

- Works together with SI to move liquids in the Lower Burner.

- Ensures that the whole organism is irrigated with the pure, extracted liquids, especially to the surface of the whole body.

- Acts as a vehicle for Kidney Yang functions, which provide energy for all body functions, while the Bladder meridian tonifies them..

- Spreads Yang throughout the body (being Tai Yang). Corresponds to the Fire of Ming Men, from where its energy is derived.

- Protects the body from the invasion of external pathological factors.

- Associated with the functioning of the autonomic nervous system through the pituitary gland, in connection with the entire endocrine system.

- Bladder Qi influences the reproductive function and the uterus.

- The Shu points along both its branches (internal and external) have a direct effect on the activities of all organs and all body functions. The internal branch regulates physical functions of the organs and the external branch regulates mental and emotional aspects.

- Together with the Kidneys it is the root of impetus, survival instinct and response to stimuli.

- Linked to the Nervous System (treating this meridian creates relaxation).

- Governs the spinal column and the physical structure of the back (BL, ST and GB keeps the body upright.)

DISORDERS / DYSFUNCTIONS

- Excessive nervous tension, hyperactivity and exaggerated reactions.

- Stiff muscles of the back, strong lower back pain, sciatica, spine-tingling, coldness and sluggishness in various parts and functions of the body.

- Pain in the inner corner of the eyes, headache or pulsations in the back of the head to the arch of the nose.

- Cystitis, urinary problems, excessively frequent, difficult or painful urination.

- Dampness in the Bladder with scanty, murky urine and difficulty in urination (due to Spleen deficiency which inhibits the effective process of fluids).

- Bladder Heat with scanty, dark urine, painful urination (due to its connection to SI, the SI can receive Heat from the Heart, originating from emotional causes, and send it to the Bladder).

- Infertility.

- Painful menstruation.

- Neurosis and paranoia (serious imbalance).

- Jealousy, suspicion, pent up resentment protracted over a long period of time.

- Eye problems.

- Sinusitis, hay fever.

- Frontal headache, occipital and neck tension.

- Nocturnal enuresis in children (caused by fear, anxiety or insecurity).

- Fears Cold and Damp (also Damp-Heat).

- Fear, anxiety.

- Insomnia.

- Tiredness.

Relationship with the Kidneys

- The Bladder receives the Qi necessary for the transformation of the liquids from the Kidney and the Ming Men.

- Kidney relies on the Bladder to move and expel a part of its impure liquids.

DAMP-HEAT

Urination problems (difficulty, burning, pain, blood, kidney stones etc.), dark urine, fever, thirst, etc.

Causes:
Prolonged exposure to Dampness and External Heat; overeating; emotional problems.

DAMP-COLD

Urination problems (frequent, urgent, difficult), heaviness and pain in hypogastrium, pale and cloudy urine, etc.

<u>Causes:</u>
Invasion of External Damp and Cold.

EMPTY-COLD

Frequent, abundant and clear urine, enuresis, incontinence, back pain, etc.

<u>Causes:</u>
Prolonged exposure to Cold (especially during menstruation); excessive sexual activity.

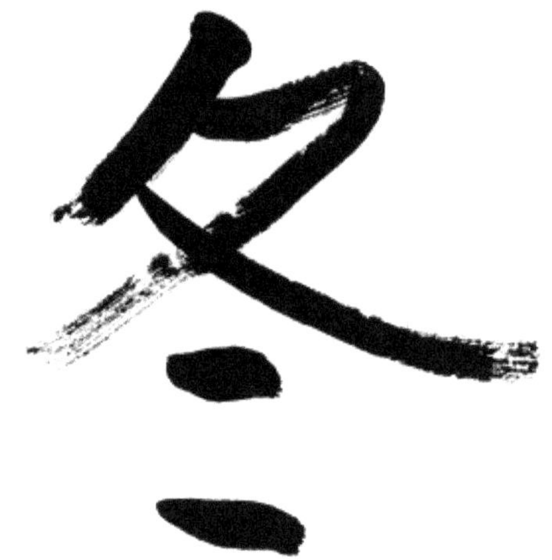

<u>BLADDER MERIDIAN POINTS</u>

BL 1   JING MING – BRIGHT EYES

Yin Qiao Mai and Yang Qiao Mai point.
Meeting point of the Bladder, Small Intestine and Stomach.

- Eye diseases, caused by both internal and external factors.

- Expels Wind-Heat (conjunctivitis, excessive lacrimation, sties, etc.).

- Clears internal Heat (eye problems from Liver Fire: redness, swelling and pain).

- In conjunction with Yin and Yang Qiao Mai opening points (KD6 and BL62) to treat insomnia or chronic drowsiness.

BL 2   ZAN ZHU - BAMBU GATHERING

- Expels external Wind from the face and removes obstructions from the meridian (facial paralysis, tics, trigeminal neuralgia, etc.).

- Benefits the eyes and calms the Liver (which nourishes the eyes). For any Liver syndrome that affects the eyes (redness, blurred vision, visual disturbance, persistent headaches around or behind the eyes, etc.).

BL 3   MEI CHONG – EYEBROW ASCENSION

- Expels Wind (dizziness, epilepsy, headaches, etc.).

BL 4   QU CHA – DEVIATING TURN

- Expels Wind and Heat.

BL 5   WU CHU - FIFTH PLACE

- Expels internal Wind that damages the Du Mai (calms spasms).

- Used in acute attacks of internal Wind (Cerebro-Vascular accident) to restore the state of consciousness.

BL 6   CHENG GUANG – LIGHT GUARD

- Expels Wind (dizziness, headache, facial paralysis, etc.).

- Benefits the eyes.

- Expels Damp (watery rhinorrhoea (runny nose), blocked nose etc.).

BL 7   TONG TIAN – CELESTIAL CONNECTION

- Important local point to disperse external and internal Wind from the head (severe headaches or facial paralysis, dizziness, cramps, etc.).

- Acts on the nose and eyes (rhinitis, eye diseases, etc.).

- Relieves spasms

- Opens the orifices.

BL 8   LUO QUE – DECLINING CONNECTION

- Expels Wind and Damp (dizziness, neurosis, tinnitus, etc.).

- Removes obstructions from the meridian.

- Raises and strengthens Liver Qi (sudden blindness).

BL 9   YU ZHEN – JADE PILLOW

- Expels Wind.

- Removes obstructions from the meridian.

BL 10   TIAN ZHU – CELESTIAL PILLAR

Sea of Qi point.

- Expels internal and external Wind.

- Stiff neck and headaches due to invasion of Wind-Cold.

- Occipital headaches.

- Purifies the brain, stimulates memory and concentration.

- Particular effect on the eyes, improves sight (especially if due to Kidney deficiency).

- Opens the orifices.

- Benefits the tendons.

- Removes obstructions from the meridian.

- Strengthens the lower part of the back.

BL 11   DA ZHU – GREAT SHUTTLE

Sea of Blood point.
(Hui) Meeting point of the bones.
Meeting point of the Bladder and Small Intestine meridians.

- Nourishes the blood, and as a result, strengthens the Ying Qi, which eliminates pathogenic factors.

- Expels Wind.

- Strengthens bones (used in children to promote the development of the skeleton and in the elderly to prevent bone degeneration - osteoporosis, arthritis, etc.).

- Fortifies tendons (used in case of contractures and aching muscles).

BL 12   FENG MEN – WIND GATE

- Expels external Wind and creates a block against an invasion of external Wind in the early stages (colds, sneezing, chilliness, etc.).

- Disseminates the Lung Qi (Wei Qi, Defensive Energy).

- Regulates Ying Qi and Wei Qi.

BL 13   FEI SHU – LUNG TRANSPORT

Back Shu point of the Lung.

- Regulates and invigorates the Lung Qi.

- Stimulates circulation and the descent of Lung Qi, which helps to expel Wind-Cold or Wind-Heat (cough, asthma, wheezing, etc.).

- Cools Heat inside the Lungs (acute bronchitis, pneumonia, high fever, thirst, dry mouth, cough with viscous, yellow sputum, dyspnoea, restlessness, etc.).

- Combined with BL43: nourishes Lung Yin.

BL 14   JUE YIN SHU – REVERTING YIN TRANSPORT

Back Shu point of the Pericardium.

- Nourishes the Heart (often used for irregular heartbeat, chest tightness and angina pectoris).

- Regulates Heart Blood.

BL 15   XIN SHU – HEART TRANSPORT

Back Shu point of the Heart.

Very important point for a variety of Heart syndromes.

-   Calms the Shen (anxiety, restlessness, insomnia with nervous origin, from Heart Excess and not from Deficiency).

-   Purifies the Heat.

-   Stimulates the brain (mental retardation, delayed speech development in children, depression in adults, poor memory, etc.).

-   Mobilizes the Blood (chest pain from Blood Stasis of the Heart).

-   Nourishes the Heart.

-   Expels Fire and Phlegm from the Heart.

BL 16   DU SHU – GOVERNING TRANSPORT

Back Shu point of the Governing Vessel (Du Mai).

-   Promotes the circulation of Blood (for heart and chest pain caused by Blood Stasis of the Heart).

BL 17   GE SHU – DIAPHRAGM TRANSPORT

Back Shu point of the diaphragm.
Meeting point for the Xue.

-   Nourishes the Blood. Used in cases of Blood vacuity in any organ (combined with the Shu point of the relevant organ).

-   Promotes Blood circulation, breaks up stasis, (moxa <u>not to be used</u>), always combined with Shu point of the related organ.

-   Facilitates the circulation of Qi in the diaphragm and in the chest (sensation of suffocation and chest pain, tightness in the abdomen, belching, hiccups, esophageal spasms, etc.).

-   Calms the rebellious Stomach Qi (hiccups, belching, nausea, vomiting, etc.).

-   Invigorates the Qi and Blood of the whole body (moxibustion and usually coupled with BL19 or BL18 and BL20).

BL 18   GAN SHU – LIVER TRANSPORT

Back Shu point of the Liver.

- Benefits the Liver and Gall Bladder. Used mainly for the stagnation of Liver Qi (swollen epigastrium and hypochondria, acid indigestion, nausea, etc.), for Damp-Heat in the LV and GB (jaundice, cholecystitis) and Liver deficit syndromes (such as Blood vacuity).

- Tonifies the Yin and Blood of the Liver.

- Subdues Liver Yang and Wind.

- Combined with BL17 to nourish Liver Blood.

- Benefits the eyes, in eye disorders caused by Liver imbalance (poor night vision, blurred vision, red, swollen and painful eyes).

BL 19   DAN SHU – GALLBLADDER TRANSPORT

Back Shu point of the Gall Bladder.

- Clears Damp-Heat in the Liver and Gall Bladder (jaundice, hepatitis, cholecystitis, etc.).

- Stimulates the descent of rebellious Stomach Qi (belching, nausea, vomiting, etc.).

- Relaxes the diaphragm (hiccups and feeling of fullness below the diaphragm due to stasis of Liver Qi).

BL20   PI SHU -SPLEEN TRANSPORT

Back Shu point of the Spleen.

- Tonifies the Spleen and Stomach and promotes the functions of transformation and diffusion of the Spleen.

- For any Spleen Qi deficiency syndrome (asthenia, loose stools, loss of appetite, swelling, bloating, stomach or uterine prolapse, etc.).

- With BL21 to nourish the root of Post-Heaven Qi (i.e. Stomach and Spleen).

- Tonifies Qi and Blood in the event of prolonged physical and mental exhaustion. To treat chronic diseases, when the patient has exhausted his energy.

- Eliminates Dampness and Phlegm (caused by Spleen dysfunction)

- Nourishes the Blood (often in combination with BL23 - with moxibustion).

- Facilitates the ascent of Spleen Qi.

BL 21   WEI SHU – STOMACH TRANSPORT

Back Shu point of the Stomach.

- As with BL20 it is one of the key points to tonify the Stomach and Spleen Qi.

- Tonifies Qi and Blood in general (often combined with BL20).

- Favours the descent of Stomach Qi (in the case of rebel Qi - burping, hiccups, nausea, vomiting, etc.).

- Dispels Dampness, tonifying the Spleen Qi and stimulating its functions of transformation and transportation.

- Eliminates stagnation.

BL 22   SAN JIAO SHU - TRIPLE BURNER TRANSPORT

Back Shu point of the Triple Burner.

- Stimulates greatly the processing, transportation and expulsion of fluids in the Lower Burner.

- Dispels Dampness because it promotes the transformation and the expulsion of impure liquids (retention of urine, painful urination, oedema in the lower extremities, abdominal masses, etc.).

BL 23   SHEN SHU – KIDNEY TRANSPORT

Back Shu point of the Kidneys.

- One of the most important points for tonifying the Kidneys in cases of any type of chronic deficiency. Indicated to nourish the Kidney Yang (with moxa), but also the Yin (<u>no moxa!</u>).

- Important to nourish the Kidney Jing (also GV4). Effective for impotence, infertility, spermatorrea, nocturnal enuresis, micturition disorders, lack of sexual desire, etc.

- Regulates and tonifies the Kidneys.

- Chronic asthma caused by Kidney vacuity.

- Through the nourishment of Jing, it stimulates the Shen, the Shen of initiative, willpower and eases depression and fear (especially effective when combined with BL52 Will Chamber – at the same height as BL 23, but on the second branch of Bladder meridian).

- Dissolves Dampness in the Lower Burner (bladder stones, cysts, lumps in the abdomen).

- Strengthens the entire back area.

- Promotes the formation of Blood, in the case Blood deficiency (combined with BL20).

- In cases of any sort of bone disease (deforming arthritis, osteoporosis, rickets, etc.).

- Nourishes the bone marrow; for symptoms of Sea of Marrow deficiency (dizziness, poor memory, tinnitus, lower limb weakness, blurred vision, fatigue, chronic fatigue, etc.).

- For all chronic disorders of the ears caused by Kidney deficiency (especially tinnitus and deafness and not for acute conditions of the ears).

- Effective for chronic eye disorders associated with Kidney Yin deficiency (decreased vision and dry eyes in the elderly).

BL 24   QI HAI SHU – SEA-OF-QI TRANSPORT

- Strengthens the lower back (low back pain, acute or chronic) and knees.

- Favours the descent of Qi in the Lower Burner.

- Regulates the Qi and Blood and removes Blood stasis in the Lower Burner (uterine bleeding, haemorrhoids, irregular menstruation, dysmenorrhea, etc.).

BL25   DA CHANG SHU - LARGE INTESTINE TRANSPORT

Back Shu point of the Large Intestine.

- Promotes the function of expulsion of LI (constipation and/or diarrhoea).

- Relieves syndromes of excess of LI (sense of fullness, bloating and abdominal pain).

- Strengthens the lower back (acute or chronic low back pain) and the knees.

BL 26   GUAN YUAN SHU – PASS HEAD TRANSPORT

- Strengthens the lower back (chronic lumbago) and knees.

- Removes obstructions from the meridian.

- Favours the descent of Qi in the Lower Burner.

BL 27   XIAO CHANG SHU – SMALL INTESTINE TRANSPORT

Back Shu point of the Small Intestine.

- Promotes the function of SI to receive and separate (abdominal colic, bowel sounds, abdominal pain, constipation, diarrhoea, mucus in the stool, etc.).
- Eliminates Damp-Heat in Lower Burner (scanty, cloudy urine, burning and difficulty with urination, etc.).

BL 28   PANG GUANG SHU – BLADDER TRANSPORT

Back Shu point of the Bladder.
Very effective for urinary disorders.

- Invigorates Bladder Qi.
- Eliminates Damp from the Bladder and the Lower Burner (dark, scanty urine, micturition disorders, bedwetting, etc.).
- Disperses Heat in the Bladder (pain and burning with urination).
- Helps eliminate kidney stones (combined with BL23 and SP9).
- Favours the transformation and expulsion of fluids in Lower Burner (combined with BL20 helps diuresis).
- Strengthens the lower back (combined with BL23).

BL 29   ZHONG LU SHU – CENTRAL BACKBONE TRANSPORT

- Cools Heat in the Bladder.
- Invigorates Kidney Qi and Yin.

BL 30   BAI HUAN SHU - WHITE RING TRANSPORT

- Facilitates the descent of Qi and disperses Heat in Lower Burner.
- Effective mainly for problems of the anus (haemorrhoids, prolapse, spasms, faecal incontinence, etc.).

The main actions of the following points **BL31-BL32-BL33-BL34** (found on the sacral foramina), is to tonify the Jing and the Kidneys. For this reason they are very effective in the following cases:

- to treat all genital disorders (uterine prolapse, infertility, vaginal discharge, impotence, prostatitis, etc.);

- to tonify the whole body in general;

- to tonify the lower back and knees.

BL 31   SHANG LIAO – UPPER BONE HOLE

See above

BL 32   CI LIAO - SECOND BONE HOLE

The most important of these four points.

- Tonifies to a greater extent the Kidneys and the Jing.

- Very effective in treating prolapse of uterus and anus.

- Effective for infertility in women.

BL 33   ZHONG LIAO – CENTRAL BONE-HOLE

- Important action on the Bladder.

BL 34   XIA LIAO – LOWER BONE-HOLE

Meeting point of the Gall Bladder and Bladder meridians.

BL 35   HUI YANG - MEETING OF YANG

- Compensates Kidney depletion.

- Clears Heat.

- Drains Damp-Heat.

Used to contact GV1 and treat related symptoms.

BL 36   CHENG FU - SUPPORT

-   Very suitable for lower back pain that involves the sciatic nerve (pain down the back of the leg), sciatica, pain in the anal region, pain in the genital organs, etc.

BL 37   YIN MEN – GATE OF ABUNDANCE

Same action as BL36.

Effective with light moxa.

BL 38   FU XI – SUPERFICIAL CLEFT

-   Removes stagnation and Damp-Heat in Lower Burner.

-   Effective in treating paralysis of the lower limbs.

BL 39   WEI YANG - BEND YANG

Lower (He) Uniting point of the lower extremities for the Triple Burner.

-   Important point to stimulate the transformation and expulsion of fluids in the Lower Burner (strengthens the Qi in Lower Burner).

-   Strengthens the Bladder.

-   For all syndromes of Excess of the Lower Burner related to the accumulation of Damp (urinary retention, cloudy urine, burning sensation on urination, difficulty passing urine, ankle oedema, urinary incontinence, cystitis, etc.).

BL 40   WEI ZHONG – BEND CENTRE

(He) Uniting point, corresponding to the Earth phase.

-   Removes obstructions from the meridian (much used for chronic back pain or acute pain with bilateral or unilateral pain, but not along the midline of the spine).

-   Clears Heat and dispels Damp from the Bladder (burning with urination, cystitis, etc.).

-   Relaxes the tendons.

-   Calms the summer Heat in acute attacks with fever, sweats, rashes, etc.

-   Clears Blood Heat (skin diseases, rashes, etc.).

-   Eliminates Blood stasis (pain in the lower legs, knee inflammation, etc.).

BL 41 FU FEN – ATTACHED BRANCH

Intersection point of the Bladder and Small Intestine channels.

- Expels Wind (pain and tension in the shoulders and back, stiff neck, etc.).

BL 42 PO HU – PO DOOR

External Back Shu point of Lung.

- Stimulates the descent of Lung Qi (asthma, difficulty breathing, coughing, pulmonary emphysema, etc.).
- Reduces pain in back and shoulders.
- For long term emotional problems and linked to the Lungs (sadness, grief, despair, worry, etc.).

BL 43 GAO HUANG SHU – GAO HUANG TRANSPORT

External Back Shu Point of the Pericardium (These points are located on the outer branch of the Bladder meridian on the back).

- Nourishes the Qi of the whole body (effective in cases of serious chronic disease, with strong debilitation).
- Tonifies the Jing (Kidney deficiency: nocturnal spermatorrhea, low sexual energy, poor memory, etc.).
- Tonifies the Lung Yin (to regain energy after severe lung disease that damages the Yin and has left the patient debilitated and with a chronic dry cough).
- Strengthens the Shen, because it tonifies the Jing, which nourishes the brain (in particular in rehabilitation after a long illness).

BL 44 SHEN TANG – SPIRIT HALL

External Back Shu point of the Heart.

- Calms the Shen (for all the psychological and emotional problems linked to the Heart).
- With BL15 for anxiety, restlessness, insomnia and depression.

BL 45   YI XI – YI XI

- Expels Wind, drains Damp-Heat.

BL 46   GE GUAN – DIAPHRAGM PASS

- Expels Wind and Dampness.

- Tonifies the Qi of the Lung and Spleen (tightness in chest, constipation, diarrhoea, vomiting, etc.).

BL 47   HUN MEN – HUN GATE

External Back Shu point of the Liver.

- Invigorates the Qi of the Liver (suitable for all emotional issues related to the Liver, such as depression, anger, frustration, resentment, etc.).

- Helps to root the Hun (coupled with BL18 it has a profound effect on one's capacity to find one's way in life, to have a purpose, a direction, dissipating the sense of frustration related to these difficulties).

BL 48   YANG GANG - YANG HEADROPE

External Back Shu point of Gall Bladder.

- Strengthens Stomach and Gall Bladder Qi.

- Treats all psychological and emotional aspects related to Gall Bladder (capacity of discernment, choice, decision, assessment, etc.).

BL 49   YI SHE – REFLECTION ABODE

External Back Shu point of Spleen

- Tonifies the Spleen, its mental aspect, the Yi (memory, concentration, learning through study, ability to make things concrete, etc.).

- Helps calm obsessive thoughts, brooding.

BL 50   WEI CANG – STOMACH GRANARY

External Back Shu point of Stomach.

- Tonifies the Stomach and helps digestion.

BL 51   HUANG MEN – HUANG GATE

External Back Shu point of Triple Burner.

- Promotes the Triple Burner functions of spreading Qi to the area of the Heart and the diaphragm.

BL 52   ZHI SHI - WILL CHAMBER

External Back Shu point of the Kidney.

- Invigorates the Kidney Qi (greatest effect when combined with BL23).
- Strengthens the back (chronic lower back pain, back pain, contractures, etc.).
- Strengthens the will (Zhi) and determination (depression with a sense of disorientation and an inability to take steps to change the situation).

BL 53   BAO HUANG – BLADDER HUANG

- Drains Dampness and Damp-Heat from the Lower Burner.
- Favours the transformation and the expulsion of impure liquids in the Lower Burner (difficult or burning urination, urinary retention, constipation, diarrhoea, etc.).
- Regulates the spread of Qi in the Lower Burner (in the uterus, in the genitals and in the urinary tract).

BL 54   ZHI BIAN – SEQUENTIAL LIMIT

- Local point for lower back and sciatica pain that extends into the legs.

BL 55   HE YANG – YANG UNION

- Expels Wind.

- Harmonises the Liver.

BL 56   CHENG JIN -SINEW SUPPORT

- Expels Wind and drains Damp-Heat.

- Tonifies the Liver.

BL 57   CHENG SHAN – MOUNTAIN SUPPORT

- Regulates and invigorates the Liver and Spleen Qi.

- Distal point, effective in the treatment of haemorrhoids.

- Distal point for lower back pain, sciatica and leg pain.

- Removes Blood stasis (menstrual pain, blood in stool, fissures, haemorrhoids etc.).

- Relaxes muscles and tendons of the lower leg (calf cramps, contractures, etc.).

BL 58   FEI YANG – TAKING FLIGHT

Luo point of the Bladder channel.

- Distal point for lumbar contractures, lower back pain and sciatica (especially if the leg pain is concentrated in the area between the Bladder and Gall Bladder meridians).

- Distal point to treat haemorrhoids.

- Tonifies the Kidneys.

- Removes obstructions from the meridian.

BL 59   FU YANG – INSTEP YANG

Meeting point of Yang Qiao Mai.
(Xi) Cleft point of Yang Qiao Mai.

- Removes obstructions from the meridian.

- Promotes the spread and descent of Qi.

-   Distal point for lumbar pain, chronic lower back pain, with weakness in the legs.

-   Tonifies the muscles and facilitates the movement of the lower limbs.

-   Strengthens the back.

BL 60   KUN LUN – KUNLUN MOUNTAINS

(Jing) River point, corresponding to Fire phase.

-   Expels Wind.

-   Distal point for back pain and chronic lower back pain.

-   Acts on the shoulders, neck and occiput, eliminating external and internal Wind (stiffness, cramps, spasms, pain, etc.).

-   Distal point for the treatment of headaches caused by Kidney Yang deficiency.

-   Eliminates internal Bladder Heat (burning sensation on urination, etc.).

-   Removes Blood stasis (menstrual disorders, dysmenorrhea with clots and dark blood, etc.).

-   Strengthens the back, muscles and tendons.

BL 61   PU SHEN – SUBSERVIENT VISITOR

Meeting point between the Bladder channel and the Yang Springing Vessel (Yang Qiao Mai).

-   Calms Wind.

-   Harmonises the Liver.

-   Strengthens muscles, tendons and spine.

BL 62   SHEN MAI – EXTENDING VESSEL

Confluent point (opening point) of the Yang Springing Vessel (Yang Qiao Mai).

-   Restores free energy flow in the Yang Qiao Mai.

-   Chronic lower back pain.

-   Tonifies and harmonises Liver Qi.

- Relaxes muscles and tendons of the external part of the leg.

- With KD6 to treat insomnia.

- Benefits the eyes.

- Eliminates internal Wind (epilepsy) - if the attacks happen during the day = BL62, if at night = KD6.

- Acts upon the spine and brain.

BL 63   JIN MEN – METAL GATE

(Xi) Cleft point of the Bladder channel
Starting point of Yang Wei Mai

- Clears Bladder Heat and calms acute pain syndromes (burning sensation on urination).

BL 64   JING GU – CAPITAL BONE

(Yuan) Source point

- Clears Bladder Heat (burning with urination).

- Expels internal Wind (seizures).

- Fortifies the back (chronic pain).

BL 65   SHU GU – BUNDLE BONE

(Shu) Stream point, corresponding to the Wood phase
Dispersion point

- Removes obstructions from the meridian.

- Cools Bladder Heat (acute cystitis).

- Eliminates internal Wind (epilepsy) and external (invasion of Wind-Cold with severe headache and stiff neck).

BL 66   TONG GU – (FOOT) VALLEY PASSAGE

(Ying) Spring point, corresponding to the Water phase.

- Purifies Bladder Heat (pain and (dysuria) burning when urinating).

- Eliminates Wind-Heat (fever, headache, pain and stiffness in the neck, etc.).

BL 67   ZHI YIN – REACHING YIN

(Jing) Well point, corresponding to the Metal phase.
Tonification point.

- Eliminates external and internal Wind.

- Purifies the eyes (blurred vision, eye pain, etc.).

- Disorders during pregnancy (premature labour, difficulties in labour, etc.) malposition of foetus.

Treat BL67 to help correct the position of the foetus in the eighth month of pregnancy (5 moxa cones on each side, once a day for 10 days).

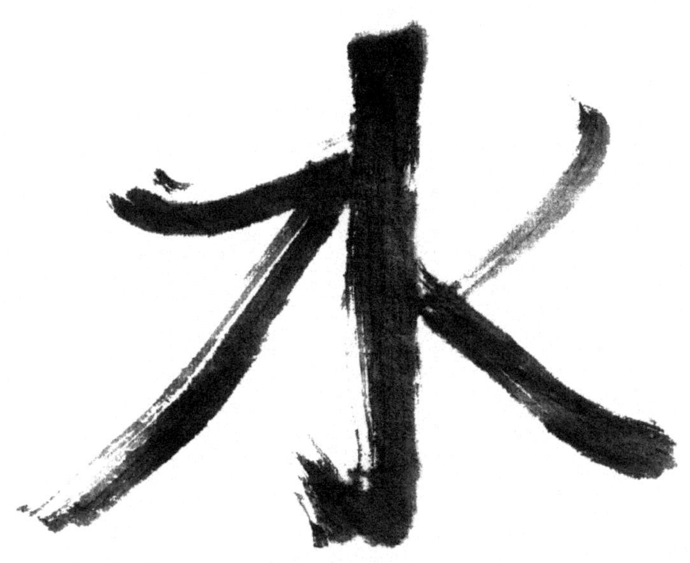

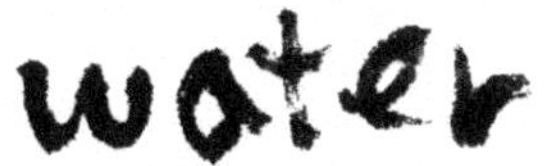

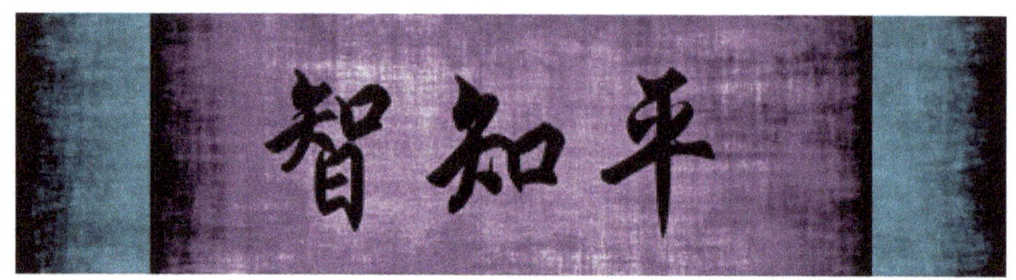

KIDNEY

IMPETUS - DRIVE

SHU POINT = BL23   MU POINT = GB25

05:00 p.m. to 07:00 p.m.

PURIFICATION OF BLOOD AND FLUIDS
STRESS
ANXIETY
ADRENAL GLANDS
HORMONES
IMMUNE SYSTEM
ANCESTRAL ENERGY
SEXUAL ENERGY AND DESIRE
REPRODUCTIVE ORGANS
PHYSICAL VITALITY
WILLPOWER
SENSE OF DIRECTION
DETERMINATION
COURAGE
MOTIVATION
INGENUITY
CAPACITY TO CONCENTRATE
SELF CONTROL
MENTAL CLARITY
MEMORY
FEAR
INSECURITY
PHOBIAS
BONES AND BONE MARROW
TEETH
EARS
HAIR

Officers who deal with energy, excellent for ability and intelligence.

FUNCTIONS

- Helps the smooth functioning of all other organs, supplying the Jing, which it preserves in the Kidneys:
    - supplies the Spleen with the heat necessary to transform body fluids;
    - assists the SI in its function of separation of body fluids;
    - provides the Qi to the Bladder for its transformation function;
    - assists the TB in its transformation function and expulsion of liquids;
    - aids the Stomach to carry out its tasks by providing the fluidity and channelling of the Jing.

- Filters and eliminates the majority of harmful residual substances that are produced by body tissue metabolism (about 80 litres of blood per hour flow through the Kidneys to be purified and transformed into nutritional substances).

- The basis of physical vitality (whereas the Heart is the basis of spiritual and mental vitality).

- Foundation of all Yin and Yang of the whole organism, the seed from which all other organs and viscera are formed. Even although Kidney is coupled with the Water element, it is home and origin of both Water and Fire (Kidney Yin and Kidney Yang or Ming Men)

- Produce marrow, fill up the brain and control the bones (three of the six extraordinary organs)

- Strongly connected to the brain (concentration, mental clarity, memory and vision). "The Kidneys are the origin of skill, intelligence and ingenuity."

- The Kidneys are involved in all constitutional and structural aspects.

- Fear the Cold and loathe Dryness.

- Closely linked to the eight Extraordinary Vessels (energy framework already fully functional at conception).

- Receive Qi from Lungs, which they gather and store for the nourishment of the whole body.

- Kidneys house the Zhi (will power): ability to translate into action the vital forces expressed by Heart Shen. Subconscious and deep desire to live.

- Opens into the Ears (large, red = good Kidney vitality).

- Governs both the Yin lower orifices (namely urethra and anus) (controls opening and closing, balancing Yin-Yang). Controls the flow of body fluids in the Lower Burner, ensuring that the correct amount of water is expelled.

- Supply Qi to the Bladder to store and transform the urine.

- Receive liquids from the Lungs; a part is expelled and the vaporised part is sent back to the Lungs to keep them moist.

- Manifested in the hair.

<u>**Supporting structure for the body:**</u>

-   origin of all the Zang-Fu (internal structure);

-   origin of the Extraordinary Vesselss (energy structure);

-   origin of the bones (physical structure).

HOUSE OF JING

<u>Pre-Heaven Jing</u>

(Yin aspect of Kidney)

-   Provides nourishment to the foetus.

-   After birth, it controls the growth, development and sexual maturity.

-   Governs reproduction (sexuality, fertility and sexual potency).

-   Material foundation for the production of sperm and eggs.

<u>Post-Heaven Jing</u>

(Yang aspect of Kidney)

Refined essence extracted from food.

-   The Kidneys store all Qi produced and not required by the body in that moment; a reserve to be drawn upon in case of need.

-   Provides the Heat essential for all organic transformations.

-   Kidney Heat provides the necessary energy needed for the last stage of formation of Blood and organic Qi.

-   Provides Heat to the Spleen to set in motion the digestive process and its function of processing and transportation of liquids.

-   Provides Heat for the metabolism of fluids and the regulation of body temperature.

KIDNEY YIN

The basis for birth, growth, development and reproduction.

Nourishes the Zang-Fu, all the energetic and physical structures of the body, and ensures that they are kept suitably moist.

Provides the material basis for the activities of the Kidney Yang.

KIDNEY YANG

Provides the Heat, the activating force of the Yin material.

KIDNEY WATER

Specific aspect of the Yin of governing body fluids, to cool and moisten the body.

KIDNEY FIRE

The Yang aspect to vaporize the liquids and regulate the amount present in the body.

- Provides Heat and energy to SI to start the transformation and separation of the pure and impure.

- Provides the basis for Bladder activities so it can carry out its functions of transformation and elimination.

- Supplies the necessary Heat to the Spleen for the digestion of food and the absorption of liquids.

<u>MING MEN</u>

A fertile meeting of Water and Fire.

The cosmic, ancestral energies that govern life.

The spark that ignites life, and whose manifestations are expressed by Kidney Yang.

A fire that must be jealously guarded and never be allowed to die out.

It is the root of the Yuan Qi (constitutional energy, deep spring/source, the Jing in movement) transported by the Extraordinary Channels with the help of the Heat supplied by the Ming Men.

The source of Fire for all the internal organs.

Heats the Lower Burner and the Bladder.

Heats the Spleen and Stomach to aid digestion.

Harmonizes sexual function and heats the Jing and uterus.

Assists the collection of Qi function of the Kidney.

Assists the function of the Heart to house the Shen.

<u>**DISORDERS / DYSFUNCTIONS**</u>

- Rickets, difficult development, fragile bones, weak teeth.

- Fear, depression, apathy, phobia.

- Insomnia.

- Tinnitus and deafness.

- Nose bleeds.

- Enuresis in children. If prolonged beyond three years of age, it may depend on great fears, traumas or the inability of the Kidney Jing to stabilize.

- Prolapse of uterus, rectum and anus (also connected to the Spleen).

- Premature senility.

- Infertility, impotence.

- Fatigue and heat in the head (dysfunction Kidney Yang).

- Oedema and cold extremities (Kidney Yin).

- Cold lower abdomen and back.

- Leg cramps.

- Pale, abundant urine (Empty Kidney Yang).

- Scanty, dark urine (Empty Kidney Yin).

- Chronic asthma (the Kidneys are unable to hold down the Qi received from the Lungs).

- Incontinence and bedwetting.

- Spermatorrhea and nocturnal emissions.

- Diarrhoea.

- Lower abdominal pain.

- Hormonal imbalances.

QI DEFICIENCY

Limb weakness, back pain, weakness in the knees, excessive and frequent urine, enuresis, loss of drops of urine after urination, premature ejaculation, spermatorrhea, chronic vaginal discharge, threat of abortion, prolapse of the uterus, oedema, decreased hearing, weak hair, asthma, palpitations, etc.

<u>**Causes:**</u>
Advanced age; constitution; chronic diseases; excesses in general (physical and sexual activity, etc.); closely spaced pregnancies; stress; insufficient rest.

YIN DEFICIENCY

Heat to the five centres (palms, soles of the feet, heart region), dizziness, fatigue, evening fever, dry mouth, bone pain, night sweats, back pain, tinnitus, deafness, poor memory, irritability, constipation, scanty, dark urine, premature ejaculation, nocturnal emission, etc.

Kidney Yin Deficiency is often the root of a Yin Deficiency in other organs.

Causes:
Stress and overwork over a long period; excessive sexual activity; long chronic disease; chronic bleeding; overstimulation of Kidney Yang (excessive use of supplements and / or medication).

YANG DEFICIENCY

Asthenia, apathy, cold feeling in the back and knees, weakness in the legs, oedema, scanty or abundant and clear urine, nocturnal enuresis, incontinence, diarrhoea, chronic lack of sex drive, infertility, impotence, premature ejaculation, poor appetite, tinnitus, respiratory disorders, etc.

Kidney Yang Deficiency is often the root of Yang Deficiency in other organs.

Causes:
Advanced age; chronic disease; excessive sexual activity; retention of Dampness over a prolonged period of time.

JING DEFICIENCY

Poor bone development, growth problems, delayed closure of the fontanelle in children, mental retardation, learning difficulties, memory loss, poor memory, dizziness, mental dullness, sterility, absence of ovulation, azoospermia, wet dreams, little or no sexual desire, brittle bones, osteoporosis, weakness of the legs and knees, lower back pain, premature aging, deafness, tinnitus, weak teeth, hair loss, anaemia, insomnia, etc.

Causes:
Poor constitution; advanced age; excessive sexual activity.

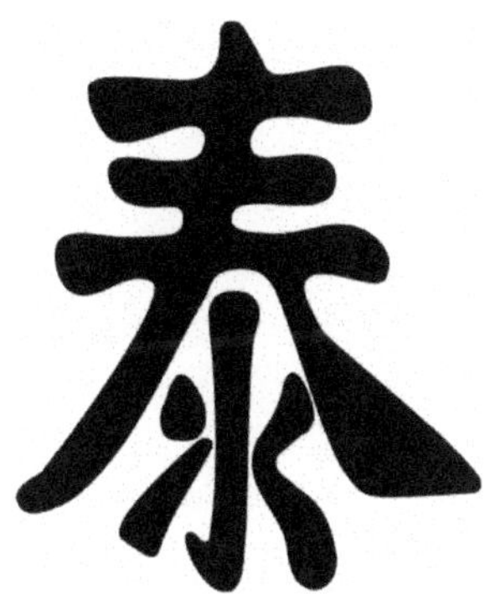

KIDNEY MERIDIAN POINTS

KD 1   YONG QUAN – GUSHING SPRING

(Jing) Well point, corresponding to the Wood phase.
Dispersion point.

- Regulates, and supports the Qi mechanism, opens the orifices, and sedates.

- Expels Heat.

- Greatly invigorates the Yin.

- Promotes the regaining of the senses in the event of loss of consciousness.

- Subdues the Wind (epilepsy, dizziness, etc.).

- Purifies the brain and calms the Shen.

- Aids the descent of the rebellious Qi (especially the Liver Yang or Wind), the Wind and Empty-Heat

- Harmonizes Heart-Kidney.

KD 2   RAN GU – BLAZING VALLEY

(Ying) Spring point, corresponding to the Fire phase.
Starting point Yin Qiao Mai.

- Clears Empty-Kidney Heat (heat in the head, night sweating, mental restlessness, thirst with dry mouth and throat at night, etc.).

- Expels Empty Lung-Heat (with LU10).

- Clears Empty Heart-Heat (with HT6).

- Strengthens the Yin Qiao Mai.

- Invigorates and harmonizes Liver and Kidneys.

- Activates the Kidney Yang (Fire) which aids digestion of food and life experiences.

KD 3   TAI XI – GREAT RAVINE

(Shu) Stream point, corresponding to Earth phase.
(Yuan) Source point.

- Noticeably invigorates the Kidneys, the Jing, the bones and the Marrow, the Yin and Yang of the whole body.

- Acts on the Yuan Qi.

- Regulates the functions of the uterus, as it is nourished by Jing (menstrual disorders, irregular menstruation, amenorrhea, excessive bleeding, etc.).

- Strengthens the lower back and knees (chronic back pain).

KD 4   DA ZHONG - LARGE GOBLET

Luo connecting point.

- Strengthens the back (very effective for chronic lower back pain caused by Kidney Deficiency).

- Tonifies Spleen and Kidney.

- Raises the Shen (exhaustion, fear, excessive shyness, depression caused by chronic Kidney Deficiency).

KD 5   SHUI QUAN – WATER SPRING

(Xi) Cleft point

- Regulates the Qi.

- Calm acute pain (micturition disorders: acute cystitis or urethritis).

- Regulates the blood in the uterus (menstrual disorders, amenorrhea, etc. Kidney Deficiency).

- Eases abdominal pain.

KD 6   ZHAO HAI – SHINING SEA

Intersection point that opens with the Yin Springing Vessel (Yin Qiao Mai).

- Important point to nourish the Kidney Yin.

- Nourishes the Yin and fluids (dry throat and eyes).

- Nourishes the Yin Qiao Mai.

- Directs energy to the eyes (chronic eye diseases, especially in the elderly suffering from Yin deficiency).

- Calms the Shen (anxiety, restlessness, etc.) and promotes sleep (effective for insomnia).

- Cools Blood (skin diseases caused by the presence of Heat in the Blood).

- Stimulates the uterus (amenorrhea, prolapse, menstrual disorders, vaginal discharge, etc.).

- Combined with PC6 helps to open the chest and promotes the circulation of Qi in the chest (for pain and sense of tightness in the chest).

- Promotes sleep.

KD 7   FU LIU – RECOVER FLOW

(Jing) River point of the five transport points, corresponding to the Metal phase. Tonification point.

- Tonifies the Kidneys (especially the Yin)

- Dissolves Dampness in the Lower Burner (oedema in the legs, swollen abdomen, etc.).

- Regulates perspiration (fever, no sweating, or excessive sweating at night, etc.).

- Coupled with SI4: promotes sweating in cases of external Wind-Cold invasion (disperses).

- Paired with HT6: stops night sweats caused by Kidney Yin deficiency (tonifies).

KD 8   JIAO XIN – INTERSECTION REACH

Intersection point communicating with the Yin Springing Vessel (Yin Qiao Mai).

- Purifies the Lower Burner.

- Removes obstructions from the meridian.

- Dissolves abdominal masses caused by stagnation of Qi or Blood stasis.

- Regulates menstrual cycle (especially Blood stasis disorders).

KD 9   ZHU BIN – GUEST HOUSE

(Xi) Cleft point of the Yin Linking Vessel (Wei Mai).

- Calms the Shen (severe anxiety, fear, mental restlessness, etc. Kidney Yin deficiency).
- Tonifies Kidney Yin.
- Opens and relaxes the chest (palpitations, tension, pain, tightness in the chest, etc.).
- Harmonizes Heart and Kidneys.
- Tonifies the Liver (to detoxify).

KD 10   YIN GU – YIN VALLEY

(He) Uniting point of the five transport points, corresponding to the Water phase.

- Dissolves Dampness in the Lower Burner (difficult, painful and frequent micturation).
- Tonifies Kidney Yin.

KD 11   HENG GU – PUBIC BONE

Intersection point with the Thoroughfare Vessel (Chong Mai).

- Connected to Kidney and sexuality (seminal losses, impotence / infertility, prolapse of the uterus and rectum, urinary disorders, etc.).
- Tonifies the Spleen, in relation to the assimilation of food (converts food into Qi and matter).
- Balances the metabolism (paired with ST30).
- Clears Heat.
- Eliminates Dampness.

KD 12   DA HE – GREAT MANIFESTATION

Intersection point communicating with the Thoroughfare Vessel (Chong Mai).

- Tonifies and regulates Kidneys and Bladder.

KD 13   QI XUE – QI POINT

Intersection point communicating with the Thoroughfare Vessel (Chong Mai).

-   Deep tonification of the Kidneys and the Jing.
-   Regulates the menstrual cycle.
-   Removes masses and blockages in the abdomen and chest.

KD 14   SI MAN – FOURFOLD FULLNESS

Intersection point communicating with the Thoroughfare Vessel (Chong Mai).

-   Invigorates the Qi in Lower Burner.
-   Regulates the circulation of Qi and Blood in the abdomen.
-   Dissolves masses and removes blockages in the abdomen.

KD 15   ZHONG ZHU – CENTRAL FLOW

Intersection point communicating with the Thoroughfare Vessel (Chong Mai).

-   Dissipates Heat in the Lower Burner.

KD 16   HUANG SHU – HUANG TRANSPORT

Intersection point communicating with the Thoroughfare Vessel (Chong Mai).

-   Stimulates the circulation of Qi in the Lower Burner.
-   Removes obstructions from the meridian.
-   Tonifies the Kidneys, Heart and Spirit.

KD 17   SHANG QU – SHANG BEND

Intersection point communicating with Chong Mai.

- Stimulates the circulation of Qi in the Lower Burner.

KD 18   SHI GUAN – STONE PASS

Intersection point communicating with Chong Mai.

- Compensates vacuity in the Spleen and Kidney.

- Stimulates the descent of the Yang.

KDI 19   YIN DU - YIN METROPOLIS

Intersection point communicating with Chong Mai.

- Cools Heat.

- Tonifies the Kidneys, Spleen and Lungs.

KD 20   TONG GU - OPEN VALLEY

Intersection point communicating with Chong Mai.

- Activates the circulation of Qi in the Middle Burner, Spleen, Stomach and Liver.

- Transforms Phlegm and Dampness.

KD 21   YOU MEN – DARK GATE

Intersection point communicating with Chong Mai.

- Cools Heat and dissolves Damp.

- Tonifies the Spleen and Heart.

KD 22   BU LANG – CORRIDOR WALK

Chest Shu point of the Lung.

- Transforms Dampness and Phlegm.

- Tonifies Lung Qi.

KD 23   SHEN FENG – SPIRIT SEAL

Chest Shu point of the Heart.

- Transforms Dampness.

- Tonifies the Heart and Spleen.

- Calms the Shen.

KD 24   LING XU – SPIRIT RUINS

Chest Shu point of the Liver.

- Tonifies the Liver and Spleen Qi.

- Calms the Shen.

KD 25   SHEN LANG – SPIRIT STOREHOUSE

Chest Shu point of the Spleen.

- Drains Dampness.

- Tonifies the Spleen Qi.

- Important point for asthma.

- Calms the Shen.

- Local point to aid circulation of Qi and Blood in the chest (Heart and Kidney Yang Deficiency).

KD 26   YU ZHONG – LIVELY CENTRE

Chest Shu point of the Kidneys.

- Eliminates Phlegm.

- Tonifies the Kidneys, Spleen and Stomach.

KD 27   SHU FU – TRANSPORT MANSION

Meeting point of Chest Shu points.

- Stimulates function of Kidney to receive Qi.

- Dissolves Phlegm and Dampness.

- Synthesises the five previous acupuncture points.

- Important point that connects Kidneys and Lungs - invaluable when the Lung Qi cannot properly descend to the Kidneys (dry cough or asthma).

- Subdues rebellious Qi.

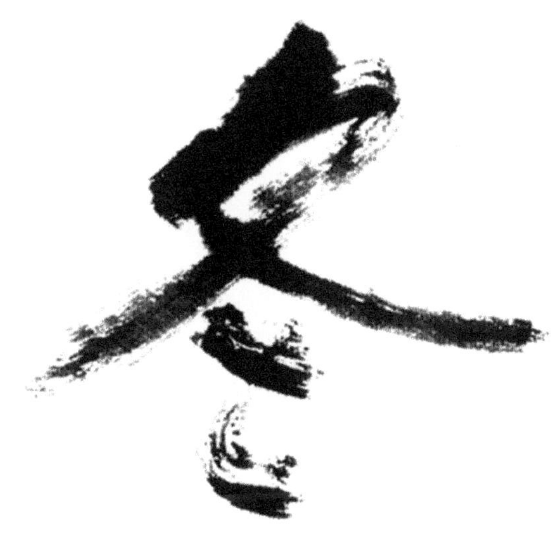

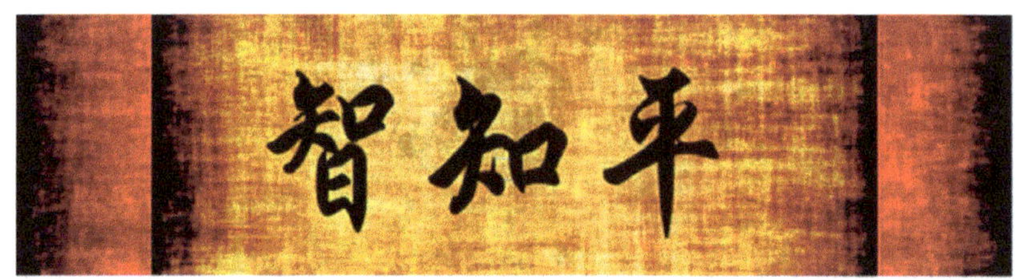

PERICARDIUM

CIRCULATION

SHU POINT = BL14   MU POINT = CV 17

07:00 p.m. to 09:00 p.m.

PROTECTION
FEELINGS
EMOTIONS
JOY
LAUGHTER
MOTHER OF BLOOD
PERICARDIUM
CIRCULATION AND LYMPHATIC SYSTEM
BLOOD VESSELS
TONGUE
SWEAT
SEXUALITY (psychological and spiritual aspect/sexual energy as an emotional experience: falling in love, sexual abuse, etc.)

Pericardium is the Ambassador and from it joy and happiness derives.

The Protector of the Heart.

<u>**FUNCTIONS**</u>

- Spreads the wishes and demands of the Heart via Blood circulation (the influence of the Shen: a sense of belonging to life and therefore feelings of joy and happiness).

- Filter and protection from harmful external influences, shock or emotional trauma, so that they do not damage the Heart (also Heat, Cold, Dampness, etc.).

- Links the Heart-Kidney (Heat produced by Kidney and spread by the Heart) and harmonizes sexuality (Kidney: physical aspect and Heart: psychological, emotional and spiritual aspect).

- Links the Liver-Heart (on the Jue Yin level), the organs most related to the emotions.

- Many points of the PC have a strong influence on the mental and emotional state, often used for relationship difficulties.

- To treat Blood Heat that causes profuse bleeding.

- Promotes the flow and regulation of the Blood in case of stagnation, especially in the chest.

- Strong, calming effect on the Shen (insomnia, mental agitation, logorrhoea and manic behaviour, anxiety and irritability, any type of shock or emotional trauma).

- Treats Heat or Phlegm in the Heart (states of delirium, seizures, coma, tongue ulcers, high fever, etc.).

- Regulates the action of the Heart in general (arrhythmias, palpitations, chest pains, etc.).

<u>**DISORDERS / DYSFUNCTIONS**</u>

- Problems with the central and peripheral blood circulation (abnormal blood pressure, swelling or feeling of cold in the body extremities, difficulty breathing and emotional discomfort due to stagnation of the Heart Blood or stagnation of Liver Qi in the chest).

- Angina and palpitations.

- Chest pain in general.

- Gastric and duodenal ulcers, heartburn (area of diagnosis of PC).

- Tendency to feel easily tired or completely exhausted.

- Stress or tension that causes restlessness and restless sleep (lack of Blood in the Heart).

- Extreme impatience, lacking the capacity to act.

- Excessive focus on work (so that personal issues take second place).

- Hypersensitivity and extremely intense behaviour.

- Demanding and aggressive attitude.

- Apparent lack of emotion.

- Carelessness.

- Vulnerability.

- Fear of contact.

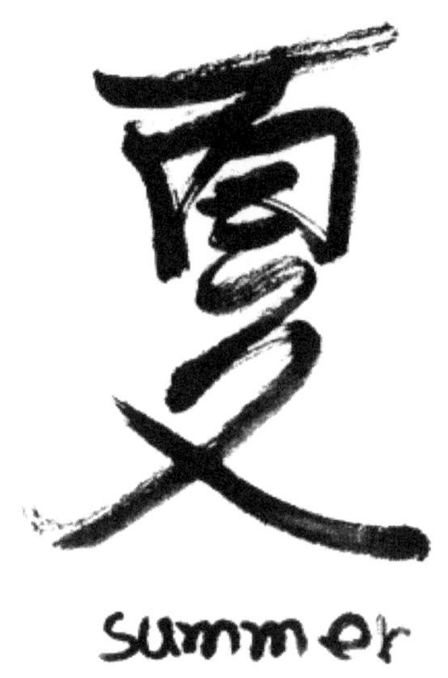

PERICARDIUM MERIDIAN POINTS

PC 1   TIAN CHI – CELESTIAL POOL

Intersection point communicating with the Kidney and GB channels.

- Expels Wind disperses and drains Dampness.

PC 2   TIAN QUAN – CELESTIAL SPRING

- Expels Wind and Wind-Heat.

PC 3   QU ZE – MARSH AT THE BEND

(He) Uniting point, corresponding to the Water phase.

- Tonifies the Heart and Lungs.

- Two important functions: regulates the intestines and cools Heat in the Blood.

- Subdues rebellious Stomach Qi.

- Clears Heat (for acute sunstroke, Heat in the abdomen, the final stages of febrile illness associated with skin eruptions and fits).

- Stimulates the descent of Stomach Qi (nausea, vomiting).

- Resuscitation point (opens orifices of the Heart to help regain consciousness).

- Cools the Blood, mobilizes and removes stasis (Heat in the Blood that can cause chronic excessive menstrual bleeding, blood clots, stagnation, uterine fibroids, etc.).

- Calms the Shen in cases of Heart Fire (excessive anxiety, palpitations, etc.).

PC 4   XI MEN – CLEFT GATE

(Xi) Cleft point.

- Regulates the Pericardium.

- Removes obstructions from the meridian.

- Being a Xi point, it blocks pain in acute conditions.

- Calms the Heart and regulates its rhythm (arrhythmia, palpitations, angina pectoris, etc.).

- Eliminates Blood stasis in the chest (great for chest pain from Heart Blood stagnation).

- Cleanses and cools Blood Heat (skin diseases, ulcers, etc.).

- Strengthens the Shen in cases of Heart deficiency (fear, lack of mental energy, excessive shyness, etc.).

PC 5   JIAN SHI – INTERMEDIARY COURIER

(Jing) River point, corresponding to the Metal phase.
Luo point of the three Yin meridians of the hand.

- Tonifies and regulates the Heart and the Pericardium.

- Important point to resolve Heart Phlegm (delirium, aphasia, coma, etc.) which, if chronic, can lead to mental illness (manic depression deep, hysteria, psychoneurosis, schizophrenia, restlessness, fits, loss of consciousness, etc.).

- Regulates the Heart Qi and removes stasis (feeling of tension and tightness in the chest).

- Subdues rebellious Stomach Qi (nausea, vomiting, etc.).

- Purifies the Heart Fire (insomnia, mouth ulcers, bitter, dry mouth, mental restlessness, etc.).

- Empirical point for malaria.

- Calms the Shen.

PC 6   NEI GUAN – INNER PASS

Luo point.
Confluence point of the Yin Linking Vessel (Yin Wei Mai).

- Regulates the Qi and Blood in the chest (tension, pain, tightness in the chest, etc.).

- Liberates Liver Qi.

- Very effective for depression, premenstrual syndrome, anxiety and irritability.

- Great calming effect on the Shen.

- Opens the chest (a feeling of tightness, chest pain).

- Promotes sleep.

- Harmonizes the Stomach (subdues rebellious Qi, epigastric pain, acid indigestion, hiccups, belching, etc.).

- Effective for neck /occipital pain, especially in women who have had a hysterectomy.

- Relieves painful menstruation and regulates irregular menstrual cycle and the emotional tension that results from either disorder (due to the relationship with the Liver and the mobilization of the Blood).

- Tonifies and harmonizes Heart and Spleen.

PC 7   DA LING – GREAT MOUND

(Shu) Stream point, corresponding to the Earth phase.
(Yuan) Source point.
Sedation point.

- Calms the Shen (more effective in women). More suitable for the treatment of emotional problems caused by the breakdown of a relationship or difficult relationships.

- Purifies the Heart Fire (important point for mental disorders such as severe anxiety, restlessness, mental confusion, manic behaviour, etc.).

- Harmonizes the Stomach.

- Expels Wind and Heat.

HT 7	**PC 7**
Both nourish the Heart Blood and calm the Shen	
Best for Deficiency syndromes	Best for Excess syndromes
Not suitable for diseases	Important for diseases caused by Heat
Slight calming effect on the Shen	More effective for anxiety and severe mania
Does not open the orifices of the Heart	Opens the orifices of the Heart
More effective in men	More effective in women, especially for emotional problems caused by the breakdown of a relationship

PC 8   LAO GONG – PALACE OF TOIL

(Ying) Spring point, corresponding to the Fire phase.

- The most important point to disperse Heart Fire and Heat in chronic or acute cases (mouth ulcers, inflammation, febrile illness, delirium, etc.).

- Calms the Shen.

(Jing) Well point, corresponding to Wood phase.
Tonification point.

- Cools Heat (for both acute and chronic cases).

- Expels internal Wind (recommended for Cerebro-Vascular attack, together with the other Well points on the hands).

- Restores the state of consciousness.

- Tonifies the Heart and the Pericardium.

- Particularly suitable for strokes, and seizures in children.

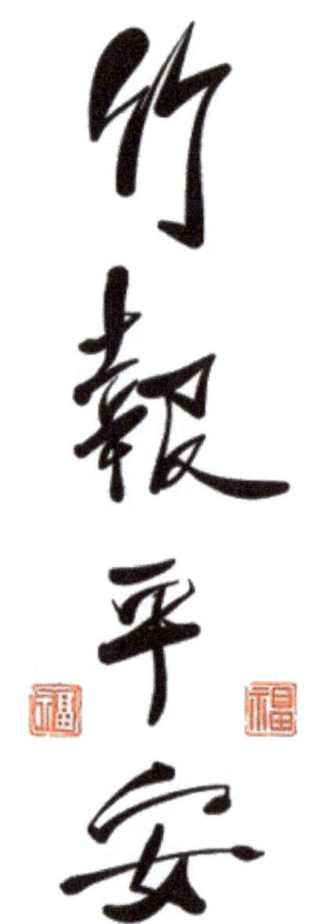

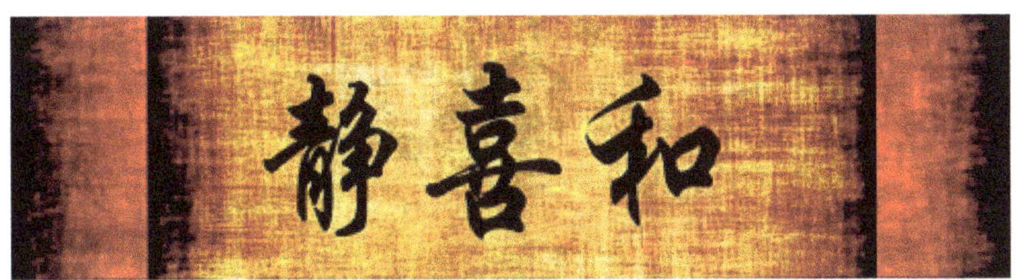

TRIPLE BURNER

PROTECTION

SHU POINT = BL22   **MU POINT = CV5**

09.00 p.m. to 11.00 p.m.

IMMUNE SYSTEM
LYMPHATIC SYSTEM
THERMOREGULATOR
METABOLIZER
ACTIVATES AND DISTRIBUTES
EXPOSURE TO HAZARD
EMOTIONAL SELF-PROTECTION
EMOTIONS
FEELINGS
SEXUAL ENERGY AS AN EMOTIONAL EXPERIENCE

Triple Burner, San Jiao is the official in charge of irrigation and it controls the Water passages (lymphatic system, water retention, blood circulation) and Grand Protector (immune system).

Works closely with the PC; it is its close associate.

FUNCTIONS

- Metabolizes, distils, diffuses; the motor that activates and makes things circulate (assisted by the force of the Kidney Jing).

- The functions of the TB involve all the Yin and Yang organs since it oversees the activation of their energies and specific metabolic systems.

- Related to Kidneys and to the process of foetal development, to the formation of a human being.

- Spreads the energy and vitality of Kidney throughout the body (PC is the Prime Minister of the Heart, and TB is the Ambassador of the Kidney: Heart-Kidney axis).

- Water passage and main thoroughfare of Yuan Qi (Kidney Jing in movement, in the form of Qi), the driving force that activates all the physiological functions of the body and provides heat for digestion.

- Activates organic transformations (food, liquids, etc.) and circulates the substances produced by these transformations (Qi, Blood, Jin-Ye, etc.).

- Governs all Qi in the organism, in particular it governs the formation and diffusion of the Wei Qi, the Defensive Qi (at the Upper Burner level), and the Ying Qi, the nutrient Qi (at the Middle Burner level).

UPPER BURNER

(Above the diaphragm) HT and LU: Like a mist.
Disperses and vaporises all purified body fluids to the surface of the body and to the whole body in the form of a fine mist (this function falls under the scope of the Lung dispersing function).

MIDDLE BURNER

(Between the diaphragm and the navel) ST-SP-GB: a fermentation chamber.
Activates the digestive process of solids and liquids and the production of Ying Qi (nutrient Qi) that the TB then distributes to all organs and viscera.

LOWER BURNER

(Lower abdomen) LI-SI-BL-KD-LV: like a "Drainage Ditch".
Transforms, separates the pure from the impure and excretes the impure.

TB and PC = paired meridians - circulation, sex and protection.

DISORDERS / DYSFUNCTIONS

- Difficulty in relationships with others.

- Being perpetually on the defensive (resulting in rigidity and tension throughout the body).

- Excessive sensitivity to environmental changes in temperature and humidity.

- Constant colds with inflammation of the lymph nodes.

- Tightness in the chest and the abdominal wall.

- Hypersensitive skin (pain, itching, eczema, hives).

- Invasion of Wind-Heat (deafness, pain in the outer eyelid, ear pain, pain behind the ears, swelling of the cheeks and sore throat – yellow or white coating on one side of the tongue; in children: red dots on only one side of tongue) – Upper Burner

- Retention of food in the stomach (connected to the function of Stomach) – Middle Burner.

- Urinary dysfunctions or disorders of defecation – Lower Burner.

- Fever and earache.

- Inflammation in the body.

- Whiplash.

- Distracted (mentally), but also clumsiness in actions and physical movements.

- Getting oneself into inappropriate situations.

- Exposing oneself to danger, both physical and emotional.

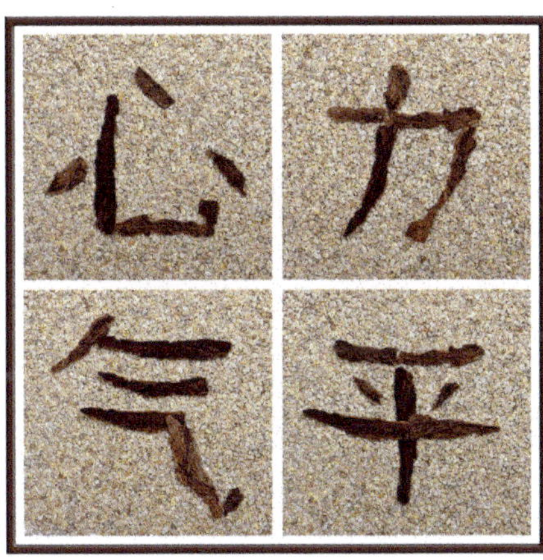

TRIPLE BURNER MERIDIAN POINTS

TB 1   GUAN CHONG – PASSAGE HUB

(Jing) Well point, corresponding to the Metal phase.

- Stimulates the transformation of liquids.

- Expels Wind-Heat (fever, sore throat, ear pain, etc.).

- Restores the state of consciousness, as it is a Well point (recommended in the acute phase of stroke and seizures).

TB 2   YE MEN – HUMOR GATE

(Yang) Spring point, corresponding to the Water phase.

- Stimulates the transformation of liquids.

- Clears Wind-Heat (inflammation of the throat, eyes, ear disorders, infections, etc.).

- Benefits the organs of sense, but particularly the ear (tinnitus, deafness, etc.).

- Removes obstructions from the meridian.

- Painful Obstruction Syndrome of the finger.

TB 3   ZHONG ZHU – CENTRAL ISLET

(Shu) Stream point, corresponding to the Wood phase.
Tonification point.

- Regulates the Qi.

- Removes Liver Qi stagnation (abdominal pain, mood swings, depression, etc.).

- Raises the Shen (recommended for depression, paired with GV20).

- Expels Wind and Heat.

- Benefits the ears (tinnitus, deafness, etc.).

- Removes meridian obstructions.

TB 4   YANG CHI - YANG POOL

(Yuan) Source point.

- Removes obstructions from the meridian (pain and stiffness in the wrist, arm and shoulder).

- Relaxes muscles and tendons.

- Clears Heat and Dampness.

- Occipital headaches (caused by invasion of external Wind).

- Stimulates the transformation and the expulsion of fluids, in the case of accumulation of Dampness in the Lower Burner (effective paired with BL64).

- Tonifies the Yuan Qi (effective in all chronic conditions, when there is a Kidney Deficiency and the patient is debilitated).

- Tonifies the Chong Mai and Ren Mai (recommended for disorders related to the Blood and Qi, such as menstrual or pregnancy disorders, painful or irregular menstruation, amenorrhea, etc.).

- Paired with ST42: noticeably tonifies ST and SP (in the case of severe weakness, debilitation).

TB 5   WAI GUAN – OUTER PASS

Luo point.
Confluence point of the Yang Linking Vessel (YangWei Mai).

- Release the Exterior: dispels Wind-Heat (fever, sore throat, night sweats, aversion to cold, infections, etc.), eliminates Cold and Dampness.

- Removes meridian obstructions (pain in the shoulder, neck and elbows, etc.).

- Benefits the ears (infections caused by external Wind-Heat or tinnitus and deafness caused by Liver Fire or Liver Yang rising).

- Temporal headaches due to escape of Liver Yang.

TB 6   ZHI GOU - BRANCH DITCH

(Jing) River point, corresponding to Fire phase.

- Regulates the Qi.
- Promotes fluid circulation and dissolves stases.
- Expels Heat (abdominal pain, constipation, etc.).

- Clears Wind-Heat in the Blood (skin diseases with rashes, shingles, hives, and itching that comes and goes and changes location - paired with GB31).

- Frees Liver Qi (removes stases).

TB 7   HUI ZONG – CONVERGENCE AND GATHERING

(Xi) Cleft point.

- Calms acute pain syndromes (being a Xi point).

- Removes obstructions on the meridian.

- Benefits the ears, temples and the eyebrow area.

TB 8   SAN YANG LUO - THREE YANG CONNECTION

Luo point of the three Yang channels of the hand.

- Removes meridian obstructions (pain in the arm, neck, shoulders and occipital area of the head).

- Relaxes the tendons, eases pain and reduces stiffness.

- Clears Heat.

TB 9   SI DU - FOUR RIVERS

- Stabilizes the flow of Qi in the head (spasms and pain in the neck and head).

TB 10   TIAN JING – CELESTIAL WELL

(He) Uniting point, corresponding to the Earth phase.
Sedation point.

- Stabilizes the circulation of Qi (Ying Qi and Wei Qi) and of fluids.

- Relaxes the tendons, stops pain and relieves stiffness (especially for elbow pain).

- Dispels Damp-Heat and Phlegm (glandular swelling of the throat and tonsils).

- Removes stagnation of Liver Qi (depression, apathy, mood swings, etc.).

- Stops excessive sweating.

TB 11   QING LENG YUAN – CLEAR COLD ABYSS

- Expels Wind-Heat pathogens from neck and back (toothache, headache, pain in the shoulder and arm).

TB 12   XIAO LUO – DISPERSING RIVERBED

- Expels Wind and Damp pathogens (pain and stiffness in back and neck muscles, headache, toothache, etc.).

TR 13   NAO HUI – UPPER ARM CONVERGENCE

Intersection point communicating with the Yang Linking Vessel (Yang Wei Mai).

- Expels Wind.
- Very sensitive local point to treat pain in the upper arm.

TB 14   JIAN LIAO – SHOULDER BONE-HOLE

- Expels Wind and Damp pathogens.
- Important local point for arthritis in the shoulder joint and joint pain (choose between TB14 and TB15 using the one most painful to pressure).

TB 15   TIAN LIAO – CELESTIAL BONE-HOLE

Intersection point of Yang Linking Vessel (Yang Wei Mai)

- Expels Wind and Dampness.
- Important local point for shoulder pain (choose between TB14 and TB15 using the one most painful to pressure)

TB 16   TIAN YOU – CELESTIAL WINDOW

-   Regulates the flow of Qi from top to bottom and vice versa (in cases of blockage of energy in the head, or trunk and limbs).

TB 17   YI FENG – WIND SCREEN

Intersection point with TB and GB.

-   Important local point for ear disorders of either an internal or external origin (infections, deafness, tinnitus, dizziness, ear infections, etc.).
-   Expels Wind, especially from the face (trigeminal neuralgia and facial paralysis).

TB 18   QI MAI – TUGGING VESSEL

-   Expels Wind.
-   Calm spasms
-   Calms fright in children (infantile paralysis, tendency to startle easily, nightmares, etc.).

TB 19   LU XI – SKULL REST

-   Expels Wind and Dampness.
-   Regulates the Qi.

TB 20   JIAO SUN -   ANGLE VERTEX

Intersection point communicating with SI, LI, and GB.

-   Expels Wind and Dampness.
-   Relieves spasms.

TB 21   ER MEN – EAR GATE

- Dispels Heat.

- Local point for ear disorders (tinnitus, inflammation, otitis, deafness, etc.).

TB 22   HE LIAO – HARMONY BONE-HOLE

Intersection point communicating with SI and GB.

- Expels Wind and Dampness.
- Tonifies the Qi.

TB 23   SI ZHU KONG -SILKEN BAMBOO HOLLOW

- Local point for eye disorders with headache and pain around the eyes.
- Local point for facial paralysis.
- Benefits the eyes (eye inflammation, loss of vision, etc.).
- Eases pain.

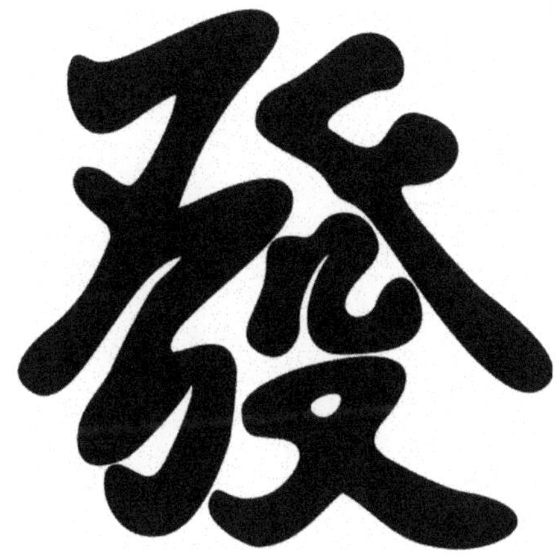

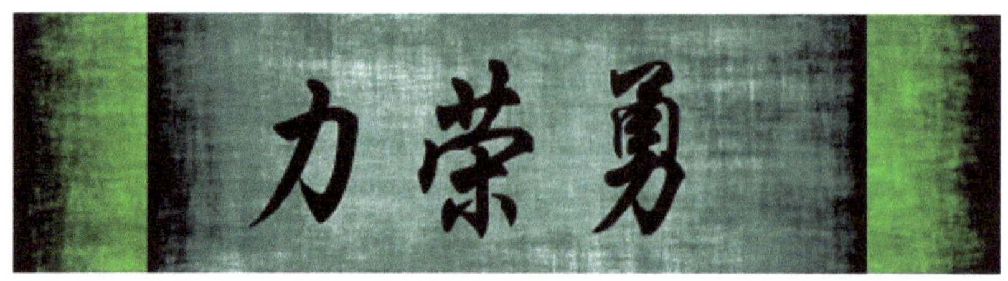

GALL BLADDER

DISTRIBUTION

SHU POINT = BL19   **MU POINT = GB 24**

11:00 p.m. to 1:00 a.m.

DECISIVENESS, DECISION MAKING
PUTTING IDEAS INTO PRACTICE
CAPACITY TO ORGANIZE
PLANNING
CAPACITY TO INITIATE
COURAGE
DETERMINATION
TAKE RESPONSIBILITY'
REFRAIN, HESITATE, TO RESIST
PATIENCE
DEPENDENCE
ADDICTION
CONTROL
RESTRAINED, REPRESSED ANGER
SHYNESS
FLEXIBILITY
COORDINATION
BALANCE
IMPARTIALITY
EXCESSIVE CONCERN FOR DETAILS
MUSCLE TENSION
MUSCLES, TENDONS, LIGAMENTS

The Officer who carries out the orders, decides and distributes energy.

<u>**FUNCTIONS**</u>

- Ability to decide and to choose (and to live means to choose!).

- Assess and make a judgment. The connection of GB with the Heart, whose task it is to discern, allows one to make informed choices on the path to personal growth.

- Stores and secretes bile (an extremely pure substance, the result of various distillations, which it receives from the Liver) and which it spreads deep into the body and, on a more material level, aids digestion and metabolisms in general.

- Sends Qi to the muscles and tendons, controlling motility and agility (the Liver sends the Blood and controls its most Yin aspect: muscle tone and strength of the tendons).

- It is one of the Extraordinary Fu Viscera and it possesses many characteristics of the organs: it does not communicate with the outside, it stores a very pure and precious substance (bile), and carries out a supervisory role over the other 11 Yin and Yang organs.

- Influences the quality and length of sleep (if you wake up early and are unable to get back to sleep).

- Supports the sides of the body and this can have a major role in postural problems.

<u>**DISORDERS / DYSFUNCTIONS**</u>

- Shyness, indecision, hesitation, easily discouraged, to give up, reluctance to take risks.

- Jaundice (when the bile is dispersed outside the Gall Bladder due to a GB deficiency).

- Waking up early in the morning and unable to get back to sleep again (GB deficiency).

- Irritability, bitter mouth, thirst, headache (Fire in the Liver and in the GB caused by long-term repressed anger).

- Postural problems (since it supports the sides of the body).

- Tension in the neck, shoulders, muscle stiffness, headaches, and migraines.

- Weak eyesight, eye disorders.

- Poor muscle coordination (tendency to be clumsy and have accidents).

- Arthritis.

- Pain in the hips, sciatica.

To relax and strengthen joints and tendons, one can treat the Achilles tendon, which, although not on the GB meridian, is the major tendon, and therefore exerts a strong influence on all the other tendons.

DEFICIENCY

Dizziness, blurred vision, high blood pressure, irritability, agitation, nervousness, sighs, startles easily, lack of courage and initiative, etc.

<u>**Causes:**</u>
Emotional problems.

DAMP-HEAT

Pain in the hips and sides of the chest, nausea, vomiting, indigestion, fever, dark, scanty urine, bitter mouth, genital eczema, yellow and foul-smelling vaginal discharge, etc.

<u>**Causes:**</u>
Excessive consumption of alcohol and fatty foods; invasion of external heat and humidity; long-term anger and resentment.

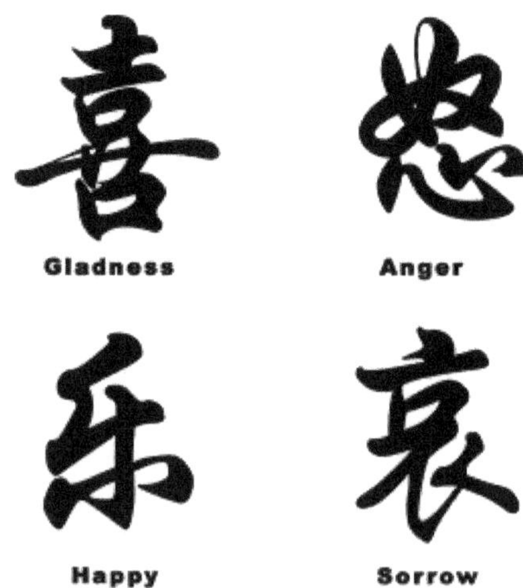

GALL BLADDER MERIDIAN POINTS

GB 1   TONG ZI LIAO – PUPIL BONE-HOLE

Intersection point communicating with SI and TB.

- Important local point for eye disorders (blurred vision, myopia, etc.) and eye problems caused by Liver Fire (dryness, redness, pain, etc.).

- Expels Wind-Heat (conjunctivitis).

- Migraines and headaches around the temple and the outer corner of the eye (caused by Liver Fire or Liver Yang).

GB 2   TING HUI – AUDITORY CONVERGENCE

- Enables Qi to flow freely.

- Important local point for diseases of the ear (tinnitus, deafness, inflammation caused by the Liver Fire).

- Eliminates External Wind (effective for otitis caused by External Wind-Heat).

- Removes meridian obstructions.

GB 3   SHANG GUAN - UPPER GATE

Intersection point with main channels of ST and TB.

- Benefits the ears (tinnitus, tinnitus, deafness, etc.).

- Eliminates Wind (facial paralysis, headache, toothache, etc.).

- Relieves spasms (epileptic fits).

GB 4   HAN YAN – FOREHEAD FULLNESS

Intersection point with the main channels of GB, ST and TB.

- Eliminates Wind.

GB 5   XUAN LU – SUSPENDED SKULL

Intersection point with the main channels of ST and TB.

- Expels Wind and Heat.

- Regulates the Qi.

- Used to treat movement disorders (convulsions and spastic movements) and speech disorders.

GB 6   XUAN LI – SUSPENDED TUFT

Intersection point with main channels of TB and ST.

- Clears Damp-Heat from the Spleen.

- Removes meridian obstructions.

- Important point for migraines affecting the sides of the head.

- For pain that goes from the ear and extends down one side of the head.

- For speech disorders, lack of motivation and willpower.

GB 7   QU BIN – TEMPORAL HAIRLINE CURVE

Intersection point with BL.

- Headache, stiff neck, toothache.

- Relaxes the jaw.

GB 8   SHUAI GU - VALLEY LEAD

Intersection point with BL.

- Removes meridian obstructions.

- Important local point for disorders caused by Liver Yang rising (tinnitus, deafness, headaches, etc.).

- Eliminates Damp, Wind and Phlegm.

GB 9   CHONG TIAN - ASSAULT OF HEAVEN

Intersection point with BL.

- Important local point for migraines affecting the sides of the head.

- Subdues rebellious Qi.

- Expels internal Wind (spasms, convulsions, epilepsy, muscle contraction, etc.).

- Calms the Shen (remarkable effect on the mental level).

- Used for disorders of movement and speech.

GB 10   FU BAI – FLOATING WHITE

Intersection point with BL.

- Eliminates Wind, Damp and Heat.

- Regulates the Qi.

GB 11   YIN QIAO - HEAD ORIFICE YIN

Intersection point with BL.

- Eliminates Wind and Heat.

- Regulates Liver Qi.

GB 12   WAN GU – COMPLETION BONE

Intersection point with BL.

- Expels external Wind (inflammation of the ear, stiff neck, etc.) and subdues internal Wind (epilepsy, convulsions, etc.).

- Regulates Liver Qi.

- Local point for headaches that occur along the GB meridian.

- For insomnia caused by Rising Liver Yang or Liver Fire (paired with BL18 and BL19).

- Calms the Shen.

GB 13   BEN SHEN - ROOT SPIRIT

Intersection point with Yang Wei Mai.

- Eliminates internal Wind (effective in the treatment of Cerebro-Vascular Attack and epilepsy).
- Very important for mental and emotional problems (for schizophrenia paired with HT5 and GB38).
- Collects Jing in the head (for this reason it is highly effective at the mental and emotional level). Paired with other points that nourish the Jing (for example CV4), it draws the Jing upwards towards the head, calming the Shen and strengthening willpower.
- For persistent and unreasonable jealousy with unjustified suspicions.
- Calms the Shen and greatly reduces anxiety caused by constant worry and obsessive thoughts (more effective when paired with GV24).
- Subdues Rising Liver Yang.

GB 14   YANG BAI - YANG WHITE

Intersection point with Yang Linking Vessel Yang Wei Mai.

- Expels external Wind; local point for disorders that affect one side of the head (facial paralysis, pain in the eyeball, frontal, one-sided headache, etc.).
- Subdues rebellious Qi (nausea, vomiting, etc.).

GB 15   TOU QI LIN – (HEAD) OVERLOOKING TEARS

Intersection point with Yang Wei Mai and Bladder.

- Eliminates Wind.
- For heaviness in the head, unclear thoughts, confusion, blurred mind.
- Regulates the Shen (rebalances mental state).
- Balances the emotions (mood swings: from euphoria to depression).
- Supports and regulates the functions of Liver and GB.

GB 16   MU CHUANG – EYE WINDOW

Intersection point with Yang Wei Mai, GB and Liver.

- Eliminates Wind.

- Supports and regulates the functions of Liver and GB.

GB 17   ZHENG YING – UPRIGHT CONSTRUCTION

Intersection point with Yang Wei Mai.

- Eliminates Wind.

- Alleviates pain.

GB 18   LING CHENG – SPIRIT SUPPORT

Intersection point with Yang Wei Mai.

- Calms the Shen (effective for mental disorders, such as obsessive thoughts and dementia).

- Regulates Liver Qi.

GB 19   NAO KONG -BRAIN HOLLOW

Intersection point with Yang Wei Mai.

- Expels Wind.

- Subdues the Yang.

- Regulates the function of Liver and Kidneys.

- Creates space for the brain (mental confusion, unclear thinking, etc.).

GB 20   FENG CHI – WIND POOL

Intersection point with TB.
Yang Wei Mai point (Yang Linking Vessel).

- Eliminates internal Wind (dizziness) and external Wind (headache, neck pain, stiff neck, etc.).

- Regulates Liver Fire and Liver Yang (one of the most important points for eye problems, blurred vision, myopia, cataract, iritis, optic nerve atrophy, headaches caused by Liver Fire, etc.).

- Acts on the ears (tinnitus, deafness and tinnitus).

- Strengthens the Marrow and nourishes the Brain (poor memory and dizziness).

- Associated with the ability to choose, awareness of past experiences.

GB 21   JIAN JING - SHOULDER WELL

Intersection point with Yang Wei Mai, TB and LI.

- Eliminates Wind and Heat (pains in shoulders and neck).

- Regulates the Qi and free flow of fluids.

- Stimulates milk production in the new mother.

- Important point for complications of pregnancy and childbirth (risk of miscarriage, miscarriages due to uterine bleeding, retained placenta, postpartum haemorrhage, etc.).

- Stimulates contractions and labour.

GB 22   YUAN YE – ARMPIT ABYSS

- Dispels Wind and Damp.

GB 23   ZHE JIN – SINEW SEAT

Intersection point with BL meridian.

- Clears Heat and Damp.

- Regulates Spleen Qi.

GB 24   RI YUE - SUN AND MOON

Mu point of GB.
Intersection point with the Spleen meridian.

- Dissolves Damp-Heat affecting GB and LV (jaundice, pain in the hypochondrium, feeling of heaviness, nausea, vomiting, gallbladder stones etc.) In severe cases pair with GB34 and LI11.

- Promotes the free flow of Liver Qi (for pain and swelling in the abdomen).

- Stimulates the functions of the GB and Liver.

GB 25   JING MEN – CAPITAL GATE

Mu point of Kidney.

- Tonifies the Kidneys (although it is more often used to diagnose Kidney rather than in the treatment of Kidney).

- Stimulates the free flow of Qi in Lower Burner.

GB 26   DAI MAI - GIRDLING VESSEL

Intersection point with the Girdling Vessel (Dai Mai).

- By regulating the Dai Mai, it harmonizes Liver and GB.

- Very important point for various gynaecological problems (irregular menstruation, dysmenorrhea, leucorrhoea, amenorrhea, endometriosis, etc.).

- Dissolves Damp-Heat (chronic vaginal discharge, vaginal prolapse, etc.).

- Synthesis of the Dai Mai, which, if malfunctioning, may impair circulation in the meridians of the legs and cause the formation of Damp-Heat.

- Effective connecting action between high-low (HT -KI). High: intercostal pain, spreading waistline, oppression, etc. Low: pain in the groin, inguinal hernia, prolapse, vaginal discharge, etc.

GB 27   WU SHU – FIFTH PIVOT

Dai Mai point.

- Warms Cold, expels Wind and Damp.

- Directs the Qi down into the Lower Burner:

In men: testicular retraction, lower back pain, tension, contractions, spasms, hernias, etc.

In woman: prolapsed uterus, vaginal discharge, menstrual problems in general, etc.

GB 28   WEI DAO – LINKING PATH

Dai Mai point.

Very similar to GB27.

GB 29   JU LIAO – SQUATTING BONE-HOLE

Intersection point with Yang Qiao Mai and Yang Wei Mai.

- Removes meridian obstructions (hip pain). Very effective paired with GB30.
- Peter Pan syndrome.

GB 30   HUAN TIAO – JUMPING ROUND

Intersection point with BL.

- Removes meridian obstructions (Painful obstruction Syndrome of the hip).
- Invigorates the Qi and Blood throughout the body and especially in the lower limbs.
- Strengthens and relaxes the tendons.
- For sciatica with pain radiating down the side of the leg.
- Drains Damp-Heat in the Lower Burner (for problems of the anus, genitals, itching, inflammation, vaginal discharge, urethritis, etc.).

GB 31   FENG SHI – WIND MARKET

- Important to expel Wind-Heat in the Blood (skin diseases, red eruptions that come and go and move, hives, etc.). Calms itching.
- Effective in herpes zoster (paired with TB6).
- Relaxes the tendons.
- Strengthens bones.
- Dispels paresis and paralysis (atrophic syndrome, cerebrovascular attack, hemiplegia, numbness, etc.).
- Strengthens the circulation of Qi and Blood in the lower limbs.

GB 32   ZHONG DU – CENTRAL RIVER

- Removes meridian obstructions (pain in the legs).
- Eliminates Wind and Cold.

GB 33   XI YANG GUAN – KNEE YANG JOINT

- Local point for pain and swelling in the knee (problems with ligaments and tendons).

- Eliminates Wind and Cold.

GB 34   YANG LING QUAN - YANG MOUND SPRING

(He) Uniting point, corresponding to the Earth phase.

(Hu) Meeting point of the tendons.

- Supports and regulates Gall Bladder, Liver, Kidneys and Spleen.

- One of the most important points to stimulate the free flow of Qi and Liver Blood (for Liver Qi in Middle Burner: pair with CV12, or Lower Burner: pair with CV6).

- Subdues rebellious Qi (nausea, vomiting, etc.).

- Eliminates Damp-Heat in the Liver and GB (paired with GB24).

- Relaxes the tendons (muscle spasms, cramps, spasms, etc.).

- Stimulates the circulation of Qi and Blood in the lower limbs.

- Removes meridian obstructions.

GB 35   YANG JIAO – YANG INTERSECTION

(Xi) Cleft point of the Yang Linking Vessel (Yang Wei Mai).

- Expels Wind, Cold and the Damp-Heat.

- Promotes the free flow of Qi.

- Relaxes the tendons (for pains along the GB meridian, with stiffness and cramping of the leg muscles).

- Removes meridian obstructions.

- Stops pain.

GB 36   WAI QIU – OUTER HILL

(Xi) Cleft point of GB.

- Expels Wind and Heat.

- Removes meridian obstructions (for all painful conditions of the meridian and the organ).

- Eases pain.

GB 37   GUANG MING - BRIGHT LIGHT

Luo point.

- Benefits the eyes (improves eyesight and eliminates phosphenes).

- Expels Wind and Heat.

- Tonifies and regulates Liver Qi.

- Directs the Fire downwards.

- Strengthens tendons and muscles.

GB 38   YANG FU – YANG ASSISTANCE

River point, corresponding to the Fire phase.
Sedation point.

- Subdues Liver Yang and Liver Fire (headaches or chronic migraines).

- Drains Damp-Heat.

- Expels Wind and Cold.

- Encourages the free flow of Qi.

GB 39   XUAN ZHONG – SUSPENDED BELL

(Hui) Meeting point of the Bone Marrow.

- Most important function is to nourish the Kidney Jing and Marrow.

- Eliminates chronic internal Wind associated with Kidney Yin Deficiency (especially in the elderly).

- Encourages the free flow of Qi in the Middle and Upper Burner.

- Transforms Phlegm and drains Damp.

- Removes obstructions from the meridians TB and GB (neck stiffness and neck pain, etc.).

GB 40 QIU XU – HILL RUINS

(Yuan) Source point.

- Removes Liver Qi stagnation by stimulating circulation.

- Strengthens the mental aspect of GB (ability to choose and decide).

GB 41 ZU LIN QI – FOOT OVERLOOKING TEARS

(Shu) Stream point, corresponding to the Wood phase.
Confluent point of the Girdling Vessel (Dai Mai).

- Dissolves Liver and GB stagnation.

- Dissolves Damp-Heat in the genital area (vaginal discharge, chronic cystitis, urethritis, etc.) and in the breast area.

- Encourages the free flow of Liver Qi (headaches).

- Harmonises the Dai Mai.

- Expels Damp (in particular for knee and hip pain).

GB 42 DI WU HUI - EARTH FIVEFOLD CONVERGENCE

- Regulates fluids.
- Drains Dampness.

GB 43 XIA XI – PINCHED RAVINE

(Ying) Spring point, corresponding to the Water phase.
Tonification point.

- Subdues Liver Yang (temporal headaches, migraine headaches, earache, etc.).

- Benefits the ears, tinnitus, ear infections, etc.).

- Dissolves Dampness.

GB 44   ZU QIAO YIN – FOOT ORIFICE YIN

(Jing) Well point, corresponding to the Metal phase.

- Tonifies Liver and GB.

- Subdues Liver Yang (headaches with periocular pain).

- Expels Wind.

- Calms the Shen (insomnia and agitation caused by Liver Fire).

- Benefits the eyes (redness and pain).

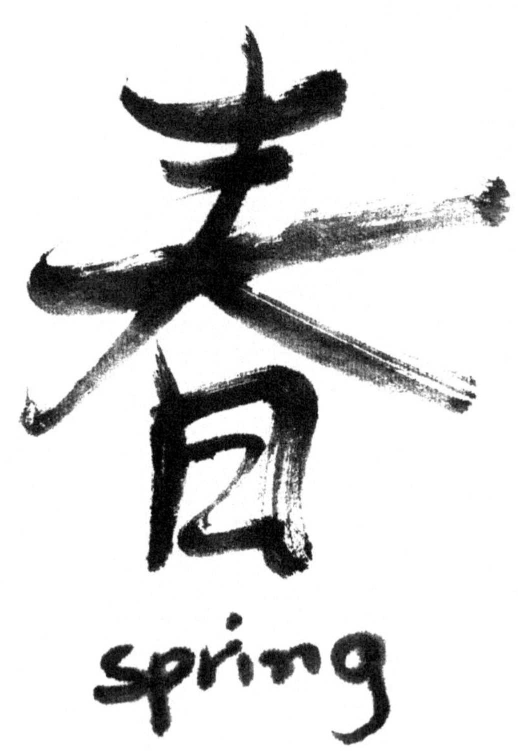

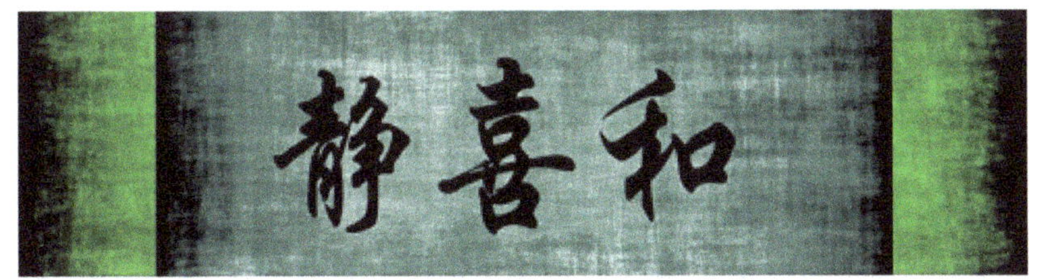

LIVER

STORAGE

SHU POINT = BL18   **MU POINT = LV 14**

1:00 a.m. to 3:00 a.m.

PATIENCE
COURAGE
CAPACITY TO ORGANIZE
PLANNING
STRATEGY
DESIGN
CREATIVE DRIVE
IMAGINATION
RESOLUTION
SPIRIT OF INITIATIVE
CAPACITY OF EXPANSION
EXTROVERSION
CLAIRVOYANCE
REFRAIN, HESITATE, RESIST
ADDICTION
DISINTOXICATION
FERTILITY
CONTROL
EXPLOSIVE, WITHHELD, REPRESSED ANGER
RAGE
ASSAULT, IMPETUOUSNESS
FLEXIBILITY
TIREDNESS, FATIGUE
MUSCLE TENSION
MUSCLES, TENDONS, LIGAMENTS
NAILS

"General of the Army, in charge of energy, harmony and strategy"

<u>**FUNCTIONS**</u>

- The Liver is the springing to life, sustained by the vital power of the Kidneys. Its dynamism and the harmonious distribution of Qi in the body are rooted in the Water component of the Kidneys.

- Ensures and guarantees the uniform and harmonious flow of Qi throughout the body and therefore affects all the functions of the Zang-Fu at various levels (emotional state, digestion and assimilation, secretion of bile, blood circulation).

- Stores and regulates the volume of Blood in the body at all times, and this serves an important function during physical activity. When the body is at rest, the Blood returns to the Liver and restores energy, and when the body is active, the Blood is sent back to the muscles, nourishing them, keeping them moist and providing them with energy. For this reason, in the case of Liver Blood Deficiency, it is very important to get adequate rest.

- Regulates menstruation (volume, flow, duration and cycle characteristics) and favours the free and harmonious circulation of Blood.

- Associated with the function of defence, immune system, protection against external pathogenic factors, in that Liver distributes Blood to the surface to nourish and protect (function also associated with Lung and TB). The Liver is the first to start the production of Wei Qi, the defensive energy that provides protection.

- Houses the Hun, the ethereal soul, closely related to Shen (imagination, creativity, design, ability to plan one's life and to have objectives, spirit of initiative, decisiveness, ability to guide, perspicacity, and enlightenment). The Yang nature of the Hun tends to make it rise upwards so it must be offset by a solid grounding of the Yin, to prevent it from re-joining 'Heaven' (panic, terror, delirious madness, madness or even death). It is the Liver that roots the Yin; a Yang organ in its manifestations, but deeply Yin in its origin (as it stores Blood, a Yin and Earth quality). So it is Heart and Blood that hold down the Hun (like a kite held by a string). A solid grounding of the Hun, closely linked to night time dreaming, will ensure that falling asleep is pleasant and rapid and that the quality of sleep is deep and restorative.

- Controls tendons and joints. Their ability to contract and relax depends on the nourishment and humidification carried out by the Blood under the control of the Liver.

- Related to vision (eyes are the sensory organ related to the Liver). Upon awakening, the Liver sends energy to the eyes; the Liver Blood nourishes and moistens the eyes and enables them to see.

- Liver manifests in the nails (considered in TCM as an 'extension' of the tendons). If there is a Liver Blood Deficiency, nails lack nourishment and become dark, ridged, brittle, breaking easily.

- Liver manifests on the left side (headaches on the left side are related to the Liver, while those on the right side relate to the GB, the left side of the tongue mainly reflects the state of the Liver and the right side the state of GB).

- The Liver detests the Wind (both external and internal).

- Liver is important, along with Spleen and Kidney, to successfully carry a pregnancy to full term (Liver meridian surrounds and penetrates the genital organs).

- Liver Qi must rise.

DISORDERS / DYSFUNCTIONS

- Anger, restlessness, impatience, intolerance, frustration and depression.

- 'Liver Fire that blazes upwards' (typical angry outbursts with violent signs of Heat in the upper part of the body: red or purple face, followed by outbursts of anger, and shouting, shaking with rage and sometimes even physical violence. After the crisis, exhaustion, empty head, sense of disgust, bitter taste in mouth, uncontrollable crying).

- Stagnation of Liver Qi, which can affect all aspects of the Zang-Fu.

- Tiredness, weakness, drowsiness or mental apathy, difficulty recuperating energy through rest (Liver Blood deficiency).

- Disorders of the genital organs (inflammation, orchitis, pain, retracted testicles, etc.).

- Sight disorders. If there is a Liver Blood deficiency: blurred vision, scotoma (partial loss of vision, blind spots), inability to distinguish colours and photophobia (aversion to light) or if there is Heat Rising: blood spotting, burning and dryness, pain, swelling.

- Difficulty in falling asleep, restless sleep, troubled by nightmares and prone to waking up during the night (disorders related to the grounding of Hun).

- Muscle cramps, contracted tendons, lack of strength in the limbs, numbness, limited extension/flexion (Liver Blood Deficiency which prevents tendons from being nourished and moistened).

- Disorders related to the menstrual cycle, such as amenorrhea (Liver Blood Deficiency), menorrhagia, metrorrhagia (Liver Blood Excess), painful menstruation, premenstrual tension, and dark, menstrual blood clots (Liver Blood Stasis).

- Eczema or psoriasis (impaired Liver function that affects the quality of the Blood).

- Headaches and neck stiffness after exposure to wind.

- Convulsions (internal Wind which is always related to the Liver).

- All disorders related to the functions of all the Zang-Fu (emotional, digestion and assimilation, secretion of bile, blood circulation), since the Liver ensures the free flow of Qi in the body, in all organs and in all directions.

- Swelling in the epigastrium, hypochondrium, abdomen or hypogastrium region (most obvious and important Liver Qi Stagnation symptoms).

- Rapid changes like rashes that appear and disappear suddenly, tinnitus, temper tantrums or in severe cases, coma and sudden collapse.

- Cracked, ridged, brittle, dry or flaking nails (Liver Blood Deficiency-unable to supply nourishment).

LIVER QI STAGNATION

Pain and feeling of fullness in the chest and abdomen, nausea, vomiting, belching, poor appetite, poor digestion, diarrhoea, feeling of obstruction in the throat, difficulty swallowing, depression, mood swings, irregular menstruation, premenstrual syndrome, etc.

Causes:
Anger, resentment, suppressed anger, frustration over a long period, preventing the free movement of Qi.

LIVER BLOOD STASIS

Irregular, painful menstruation with dark menstrual blood that is full of clots, purplish skin and nails, dry skin, constant and fixed abdominal pains, abdominal masses, vomiting of blood, etc.

Causes:
Always linked to emotional problems, it is often the result of a long-term stagnation of Qi.

LIVER BLOOD DEFICIENCY

Pale face, vertigo, tinnitus, limb numbness, blurred vision, muscle spasms, cramps, brittle nails, dry skin, insomnia, sleep disturbed by many dreams, very scanty or no menstruation, etc.

Causes:
Severe bleeding; chronic menorrhagia; diet poor in nutrients; Qi or Kidney Jing deficiency.

LIVER YIN DEFICIENCY

Dizziness, light-headedness, headache, blurred vision, dry eyes, hot flushes, irritability, night sweats, etc.

Causes:
May result from a Kidney Yin deficiency; excessive physical and/or sexual activity; chronic menorrhagia.

LIVER YANG DEFICIENCY

Acute pain in the lower abdomen, painful menstruation, inguinal hernia, scrotal pain, etc.

Causes:
Invasion of external Cold.

LIVER YANG RISING

Headache with pain that radiates to the temples and eyes, swollen face and eyes, high blood pressure, palpitations, amnesia, dizziness, tinnitus, deafness, dry mouth, irritability, anger, insomnia, etc.

Causes:
Anger, resentment, frustration over a long period of time; anxiety and fright.

LIVER FIRE RISING

Irritability, outbursts of anger, mental instability, violent headache, dizziness, red face and eyes, tinnitus, insomnia, nightmares, dry, bitter mouth, herpes zoster, constipation with dry stools, bleeding in the upper part of the body (epistaxis, haemoptysis - coughing up blood), dark urine, etc.

Causes:
Repressed anger, frustration, and resentment over a long period of time; prolonged stagnation of Qi; excessive alcohol consumption, smoking, excessive consumption of fried or fatty foods.

EXTREME HEAT GENERATING WIND

High fever with tremors, convulsions, thirst, stiff neck, eyes rolled back, opisthotonos (muscle spasms causing backward arching of head, neck and spine), coma, etc.

Causes:
External Heat that penetrates the Blood.

WIND FROM YANG RISING

Dizziness, headache, sudden loss of consciousness, hemiplegia, convulsions, slurred speech, twitching, numbness, deviation of the mouth and eyes, etc.

Causes:
Liver and Kidney Yin Deficiency; anger, frustration, resentment, etc.

WIND FROM LIVER BLOOD DEFICIENCY

Numbness of the limbs, cramp in hands and feet, muscle tremors, dizziness, etc.

Causes:
Chronic Liver Blood Deficiency.

DAMP HEAT OF LIVER AND GALL BLADDER

Fever, pain in the chest and hips, feeling of fullness, bitter mouth, nausea, vomiting, poor appetite, scanty, dark urine, redness and itching in genitals, vaginal discharge, etc.

Causes:
Spleen Qi Deficiency (excessive consumption of fatty foods, sweets, alcohol, etc.); stagnation of Liver Qi; external Damp-Heat.

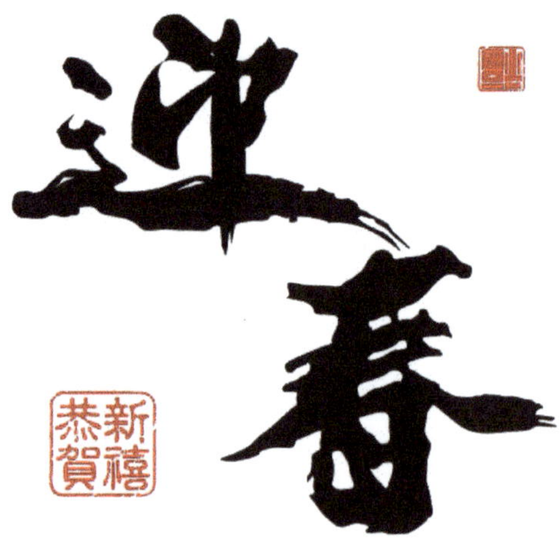

LIVER MERIDIAN POINTS

LV 1   DA DUN – LARGE PILE

(Jing) Well point, corresponding to Wood phase.

- Exerts a decisive influence on the Lower Burner.

- Regulates the menstrual cycle.

- Stops uterine bleeding caused by Blood Heat (not recommended if caused by Qi deficiency).

- Dissolves Damp-Heat in Lower Burner (difficult urination, urine retention, swollen scrotum, scrotal itching, vaginal or vulvar itching).

- Encourages the free flow of Liver Qi, especially in the Lower Burner.

- Restores the state of consciousness (as do many Well points). Used in the acute phases of Cerebrovascular accident.

LV 2   XING JIAN – MOVING BETWEEN

(Ying) Spring point, corresponding to the Fire phase.
Sedation point.

- Drains Liver Fire (bitter mouth, thirst, flushed face, headache, sleep disturbed by dreams, scanty, dark urine, constipation, red eyes, red tongue with thick, yellow coating).

- Subdues Liver Yang (migraine caused by Liver Yang rising).

- Expels internal Wind (epilepsy and seizures in children).

- Treats coughs caused by Liver Fire attacking the Lungs and obstructing the chest (usually accompanied by pain below the ribs).

LV 3   TAI CHONG – SUPREME SURGE

(Shu) Stream point, corresponding to the Earth phase.
(Yuan) Source point.

- Sinks Liver Yang and Liver Fire (migraines caused by Liver Yang rising).

- Expels internal Wind and calm spasms and muscle cramps.

- Expels Wind from the face (facial palsy and tics). Paired with LI4.

- Calms the Shen (calms patients who are extremely tense, prone to angry outbursts, or with feelings of great frustration and suppressed anger or in cases of nervous tension caused by stress). Paired with LI4 increases the effect.

- Encourages the free flow of Liver Qi and Blood.

- Highly recommended to calm the Liver in syndromes of Excess.

LV 4   ZHONG FENG – MOUND CENTRE

(Jing) River point, corresponding to the Metal phase.

- Encourages the free flow of Liver Qi in the Lower Burner (genital area and urinary tract).

LV 5   LI GOU – WOODWORM CANAL

Luo point.

- Acts, in particular, on the genital area and urinary tract.

-   Dissolves Damp-Heat in the Lower Burner (vaginal discharge or cloudy urine).

-   For Liver Qi Stagnation in the throat (feeling of a lump in the throat, difficulty swallowing).

LV 6   ZHONG DU - CENTRAL METROPLOLIS

(Xi) Cleft point.

-   Tonifies and regulates the Blood.

LV 7   XI GUAN – KNEE JOINT

-   For Painful Obstruction Syndrome of the knee, particularly when caused by Wind, wandering pain, and when the pain is on the inner side of the knee.

LV 8   QU QUAN – SPRING AT THE BEND

(He) Uniting point, corresponding to the Water phase.
Tonification point.

-   Dissolves Damp-Heat and Damp-Cold in the Lower Burner (urinary retention, cloudy urine, burning with urination, vaginal discharge, vulvar itching).

-   Nourishes Liver Blood.

-   Tonifies the Liver Yin.

-   Relaxes the tendons.

-   Benefits the Bladder.

LV 9   YIN BAO – YIN BLADDER

-   Encourages the free flow of Qi and Blood in the Lower Burner.

LV 10   ZU WU LI – FOOT FIVE LI

- Drains Dampness.

- Tonifies the Spleen.

LV 11   YIN LIAN - YIN CORNER

- Regulates the Blood.

- Benefits childbirth (difficult or delayed childbirth.)

LV 12   JI MAI - URGENT PULSE

- Eliminates Wind.

- Tonifies the Liver and Kidney Yin.

LV 13   ZHANG MEN – CAMPHORWOOD GATE

Mu point of the Spleen.
(Hui) Meeting point for all the Viscera (Fu Organs).

- Used in all cases of stagnation of Liver Qi that invades the Stomach and Spleen.

- Encourages the free flow of Liver Qi and eliminates stasis.

- Eliminates the retention of food.

- Benefits Stomach and especially the Spleen.

LV 14   QI MEN – CYCLE GATE

Mu point of the Liver.
Yin Wei Mai point.
Intersection point with GB and Yin Linking Vessel.

- Encourages the free flow of Liver Qi.

- Acts on the stomach (nausea, vomiting, swelling and pain, burping, etc.).

- Harmonizes the Liver and Stomach Qi.

- Cools Heat in the Blood.

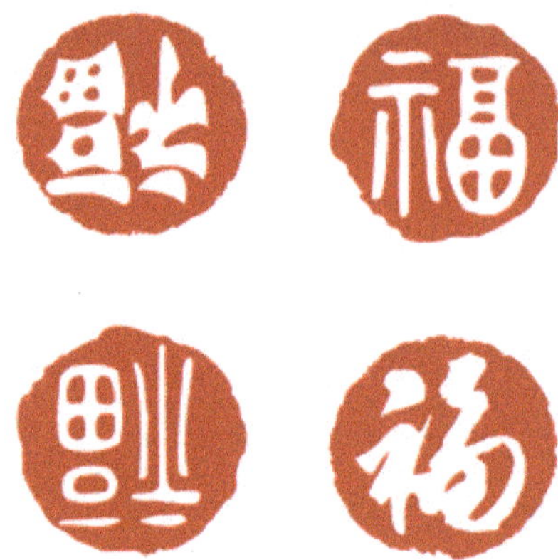

EXTRAORDINARY VESSELS (Qi Jing Ba Mai)

Together with the six Extraordinary Fu Viscera, they represent the energy network that develops and is activated at the moment of conception and which influences one's experiences and relationships.

The first structures to develop within the embryo are the Extraordinary Fu Viscera (Marrow, Brain, Bone, Uterus, Vessels, Gall Bladder); then follow the organs, the viscera (with all conformations related to them) and, in parallel, the 8 Extraordinary Vessels, from which all the other energy pathways are formed.

The Extraordinary Vessels represent the constitutional aspects of the individual, his energetic framework; for this reason they are mainly related to the Pre-Heaven Qi (Shen, Jing, Extraordinary Structures).

They especially favour the spiritual evolution of the individual.

In classical texts they are compared to lakes, reservoirs of energy that can absorb energy from the Principal Meridians (considered rivers) or transfer it when needed.

Like all the secondary channels, they also carry out the role of defence against external factors, but being more related to the deep-rooted constitution of the individual they are not particularly influenced by these external factors.

The Extraordinary Vessels carry the Yuan Qi (constitutional energy), the most vital energy (Jing in motion) and they are closely linked to the trunk, where our life essence resides (the Ming Men). This demonstrates their close relationship with the Kidneys.

Apart from the Du Mai (Governing Vessel) and Ren Mai (Conception Vessel), the Extraordinary Vessels do not have any of their own points.

They play a determining role during gestation. <u>In pregnancy</u> the treatment of the Extraordinary Vessels also serves to activate the same vessels in the baby.

They are divided into:

1ST GENERATION

CHONG MAI – REN MAI - DU MAI – DAI MAI

- Related to Pre-Heaven, at conception.
- The potential for life that prepares the passage from the Pre-Heaven to Post-Heaven.
- The first to be formed in the foetus (creating the 'energetic trunk').
- Creates the conditions for one to realize one's potential in life.
- All the structural problems of a hereditary nature.
- Ren Mai (CV) and Du Mai (GV) have their own points whereas Chong Mai and Dai Mai share points with the 12 Principal Meridians.

2ND AND 3RD GENERATION

YIN / YANG WEI MAI -   YIN / YANG QIAO MAI

- The entry of the individual into the Post-Heaven.
- Activation in life of this possibility.
- Preparation for the impact with the world, making one's way in the world.
- Connection between Pre-Heaven and Post-Heaven.
- The creation of the pre-conditions for one to realize one's potential.
- Related to constitutional issues arising from utilisation of the Jing and Yuan Qi and therefore to the process of existence, growth, and ageing.

<u>CHONG MAI</u> (Penetrating Vessel) - Sea of Blood

- A vessel in the centre of the trunk, which begins its development at the Ming Men point (VG4).
- Represents precisely the power of the energy of life, the explosion of life.
- Verticalization, expansion.
- Through this channel vitality is enhanced.
- The primordial life force.
- The Jing in motion.
- A very profound aspect of change

CHANGE -TRANSFORMATION

<u>REN MAI</u> (Conception Vessel) - Sea of Yin

- Caring for oneself, self-esteem
- Take responsibility for one's life.
- Associated with the mother figure that gives nourishment, care, attention.
- Concerns all Yin aspects and is activated in all Yin situations (pregnancy, menstruation, menopause, depression, hospitalization for illness, childbirth, breastfeeding, etc.).

CARING FOR ONESELF

<u>DU MAI</u> (Governing Vessel) - Sea of Yang

- Ability to stand erect and live life to the full. Ability to go one's own way.
- Evolution, self-assertion, self-improvement, self-determination, have a direction in life.
- Sense and commitment associated with what we do.
- Associated with the father figure who gives direction.
- Ability to achieve what one desires.
- Problems related to the spine (scoliosis).

EVOLUTION - ASSERTIVENESS

<u>DAI MAI</u> (Girdling Vessel)

- Union, cohesion, holding together.

- Communicate, aid communication.

- Connection.

- Contains, but also promotes communication and flow of energy (for this reason, like a belt, it should not be too tight or too loose).

- <u>NOT</u> to be treated during pregnancy.

COHESION - COMMUNICATION

<u>WEI MAI</u>

- First activation of the vital energy towards the Post-Heaven.

- Links the various phases of life, the stages (birth, growing up, maturing, growing old, death).

- Treated when there is transitional difficulties with these stages of development (teenagers with pimples/acne, depression in the elderly, etc.)

- Helps greatly in cases of terminal illness, as a way towards death (draws on resources needed in order to die well, to live well this final transition).

CONNECTION

<u>YIN WEI MAI</u> (Yin Linking Vessel)
- Structural aging.

- Collects and distributes Kidney Yin.

- Depletion of Jing.

- Finds and draws on the resources efficiently.

<u>YANG WEI MAI</u> (Yang Linking Vessel)
- Aging related to the ability to act and choose (GB) and this therefore includes the ability to renounce.

- Implementation of power (as our options and choices diminish, leaving fewer and fewer, and, as is the case in the aging process, one tends to become more mentally inflexible).

- Expend one's opportunities for choice.

QIAO MAI

- "Rise up on the heels" to see far and to move in the world.

- The journey of personal growth (strongly linked to meditative practices).

- Knowing the world to know oneself and vice versa. Gain and internalise experiences.

- Being in the here and now, looking outside and accepting the world (Yang Qiao) and oneself (Yin Qiao).

ACCEPTANCE - AWARENESS

YIN QIAO MAI (Yin Springing Vessel)

- Introspection (in relation to what happens outside) and see how we respond to the facts of the outside world.

- Self-awareness.

- Being in the world in the here and now.

- Self-acceptance and self-confidence.

- Disorders: mistrust in oneself, depression.

YANG QIAO MAI (Yang Springing Vessel)

- Ability to look at the world and accept it for what it is.

- Experience of contact with the outside world.

- Disorders: introversion, rejection of the world, detachment.

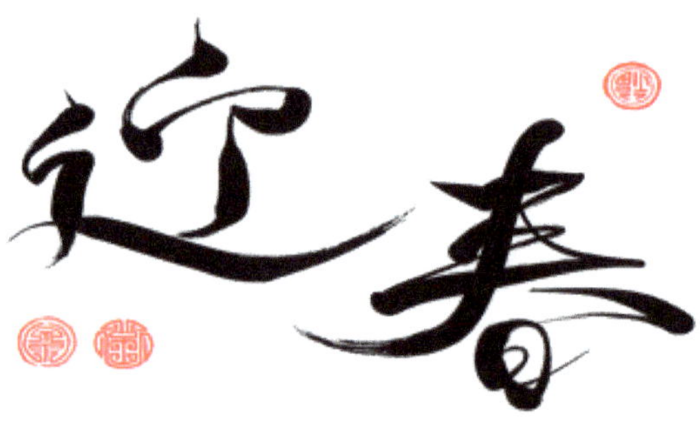

VESSELS	KEYWORD	DISORDER
CHONG MAI	CHANGE	physical and mental steadiness
DU MAI	SELF-AFFIRMATION	weak-willed, dictatorial
REN MAI	SELF CARE	carelessness, perpetually dissatisfied, over-dependence (narcissism)
DAI MAI	COHESION	dispersion, blockage
WEI MAI	CONNECTION	
Yin	to distribute Kidney Yin	keep inside
Yang	to choose	inflexibility
QIAO MAI	ACCEPTANCE	
Yin	of themselves	self-doubt, depression
Yang	of the world	rejection of the world

It takes about eight years for the ordinary energy pathways to develop and become operational. When these are fully active the Extraordinary Vessels delegate functions to the Principal Meridians and therefore no longer operate automatically, but as a support and as a continuous recreation and connection with the deep ancestral energies.

The activation of the Extraordinary Vessels (through specific exercises such as Qi Gong, Tai Qi, Yoga, etc.) can help reduce the consumption of Jing.

These vessels have a supply and regulatory function compared to the Principal Meridians (the Nei Jing describes the Main Channels as rivers and the Extraordinary Vessels as lakes).

OPENING POINTS

Unlike the Principal Meridians, the energy conveyed by the Extraordinary Vessels, (Yuan Qi), flows slowly and deeply, so it is not always active and noticeable on the surface. To gain access to these vessels the doors must first be unlocked to allow entry, the energy can then be engaged, made perceptible and therefore be treated.

From the Post-Heaven world these points allow us to access our ancestral energies, the Pre-Heaven world.

Most of these opening points are Luo points (large points connecting to the depths, because they are closely related to the Blood, which also carries all our memories and experiences).

These are points to touch, to explore, until they reveal themselves (they help to connect with a person's most inner self).

<u>LUO POINTS:</u>   SP4 - PC6 - TB5 - LU7

Connected at a deep level (Blood, Interior, Ying Qi)

<u>SHU STREAM POINTS:</u>   SI3 - GB41

Their function is to connect the interior with the exterior

<u>WATER POINTS:</u>   KD6 - BL62

Ankle area, connected to Water. Connection with the Yuan Qi

GONG SUN   SP 4 – Grandfather Grandson

<u>Gong</u>: maternal grandfather, highest level in the family hierarchy, power, impartiality, authority, the source of wisdom.

<u>Sun</u>: Grandson, descending, bud, connection.

- Bequeath and transmit life.
- Luo point (connection between exterior and interior, with depth).
- Opens Chong Mai.

ZHAO HAI   **KD 6 – Shining Sea**

Hai: the sea, large lake, multitude.
Zhao: shining sunlight, illuminate, reflect.

Point connected to the meditative practices; puts us in touch with our inner self.

The outside world becomes a mirror; to look at the outside world, one can see

inside oneself.

-   Opens Yin Qiao.

SHEN MAI   **BL62 – Extending Vessel**

Shen: spirit.

-   Name of the ninth hour of the day (15-17 Water).

-   Extend, stretch, stand up, rise up (spiritually).

-   Opens Yang Qiao.

N.B The ideogram in this case is different from the other Shen.

Shen = spirit: the influx that comes down from the heaven and

Lin = the individual spirit that shines forth (from the eyes).

ZU LIN QI   **GB41 – Foot Overlooking Tears**

Place that collects and governs the turbid fluids in the lower part of the body.

Zu: foot (which is below).
Qi: tears (cry), water, gathering place of turbid waters.
Lin: governing, controlling, inspecting, overseeing, honouring a guest.

To eliminate all accumulations of turbidity, stagnation in the Lower Burner, including
constipation (but not if caused by a Qi Deficiency which is frequent in the elderly),
leucorrhoea, cystitis, diarrhoea, candida, stagnation of Dampness (fibroids, cellulite, etc.).

-   Opens Dai Mai.

NEI GUAN   **PC6 – Inner Pass**

Nei: internal, inside.
Guan: gate, step, border, shut.

It gives access to something precious that is guarded.

- Luo point.
- Opens Yin Wei.

WAI GUAN   **TB5 – Outer Pass**

Protection and communication with the outside.

- Luo point.
- Opens Yang Wei.

LIE QUE   **LU7 – Branching Cleft**

Lie: divide, segment, separate.
Que: basin (water collection), place empty, hollow, incomplete.

Reservoir where the Qi from the Lungs is gathered and divided between the12 Principal Meridians.

The energy of the morning is collected in the Lung to be distributed to the various channels. LU7 is the point where this subdivision and diffusion takes place.

Opening point of Ren Mai, which is responsible for regulating individual growth, ensuring the maternal aspect of nutrition, division and distribution according to need.

- Difficulties with breastfeeding and let down of milk.
- Lung is closely related to memories of the past (including past lives), to forgiveness.
- Luo point.
- Opens Ren Mai.

HOU XI   **SI3 – Back Ravine/ Back Stream**

Hou: rear, further, next.
Xi: ravine, the river that runs between the gorges.

Opening point of Du Mai; it is like a deep river that carries the energy from the marrow to the brain ('sea of marrow') embedded in the branches of Bladder.

- (Shu) Stream point

- Tonification point for SI (Tae Yang).

- Opens Du Mai.

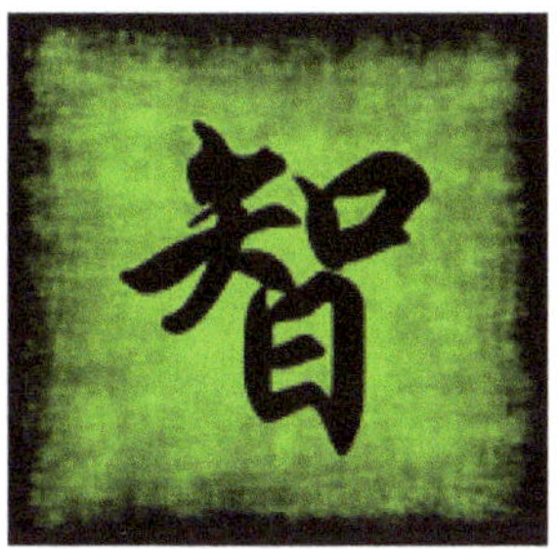

<u>COUPLED POINTS</u>

They are used to connect the generations (one from the first and the other from the second or third), the Yin with the Yin and the Yang with the Yang, or in order to create a specific energetic effect, in relation to the characteristics of the paired channels.

CHONG MAI	**YIN WEI**
SP4	**PC6**
Father	Mother

<u>Blood</u>

- produces it	- spreads it
- gives it power	- activates the power
- the seed	- the stages of life
	- pregnancy of nine months

Activates the profound capacity for transformation and change by dissemination. Spreading of Pre-Heaven energy to Post-Heaven.

DU MAI	**YANG QIAO**
SI 3	**BL62**
Groom	Bride

<u>Tai Yang</u>

- give life structure	- manage life relationships
- make sense, give life a direction	- look at the outside world
- aim high, self-affirmation	- manage relations with the outside world

Stimulates the development and spiritual growth through the acceptance of life experiences.

Promotes the ability to accept what comes to us from the outside and, through this, to evolve.

DAI MAI	**YANG WEI**
GB41	**TB5**
Son	Daughter

<u>Shao Yang</u>

- ability to connect and to communicate	- linked to activity
- unlock fixations	- to live life, make one's way in it
- unity and cohesion	

Helps to choose, to let go of what is not needed.

Brings a sense of unity and cohesion in how you act and move in the world, which is to choose and so to live.

Being in the here and now but without being fixated on something.

REN MAI	**YIN QIAO**
LU7	**KD6**
The host	The guest

- welcomes the world	- accepts the hospitality of the world
- takes care of himself	- self esteem
	- acceptance of self

Stimulates the ability of inner development by taking responsibility for one's own life, accepting oneself.

The ability to look inwards.

OTHER COMBINATIONS

REN MAI	**DU MAI**
LU7	**SI3**
Sea of Yin	Sea of Yang

Activation, communication and deep and global rebalancing of all the Yin and Yang.

DAI MAI	**CHONG MAI**
GB41	**SP4**
- horizontal and circular movement and containment	- vertical thrust

Stimulates vitality by offering containment or a better fluidity.

| **YIN WEI** | **YANG WEI** |
| PC6 | TB5 |

Global effect on the functions of connection between the various parts of the body.

Inherent problems relating to the transitional stages of life (childhood, adolescence, adulthood, old age, death, moving house, change of job, relationships, etc.).

Connection between the inner world and outer world.

| **YIN QIAO** | **YANG QIAO** |
| KD6 | BL62 |

Acceptance of self and of the world.

Balancing activity/rest (sleeping/waking).

Unresolved, unabsorbed trauma, paresis (also Wei Mai).

Emotional blocks associated with changes that are difficult to implement.

CHONG MAI	**REN MAI**
SP4	LU7
Sea of Blood	Sea of Yin

Nourishes the Blood.

Activates all the Yin, including the Blood (Xue).

Very powerful for problems associated with femininity.

For women who fail to conceive.

YIN QIAO	**YIN WEI**
KD6	**PC6**
Self –acceptance	Transition stages

Ability to accept oneself in the transitional stages of life and take what we need in order to evolve.

YANG WEI	**YANG QIAO**
TB5	**BL62**
Move in the world	Accept the world

Ability to move in a world that we accept.

DU MAI	**DAI MAI**
SI 3	**GB 41**
Direction, support	Cohesion, containment, sense of limits

CHONG MAI - REN MAI - DU MAI – DAI MAI

Works globally on Pre-Heaven energies.

YIN and YANG WEI -YIN and YANG QIAO

Connection and acceptance of the inner self to relate and interact with the world.

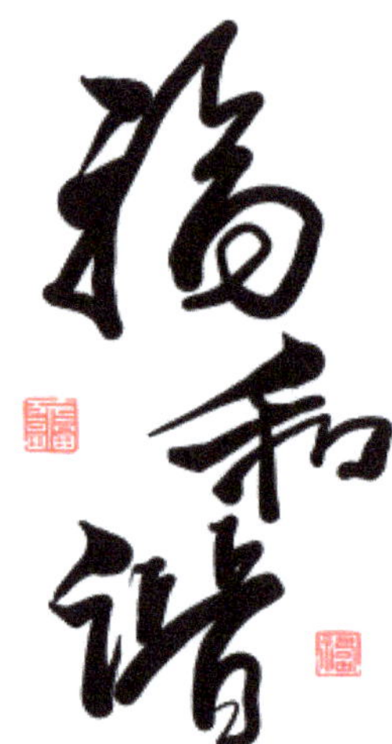

Over and above the opening points, each Extraordinary Vessel has a Start point and an End point; the second and third generation vessels have also got a Release point.

START POINT

The Start point of the vessel does not always coincide with the Opening point.

It indicates to which deep energy the Extraordinary Vessel is connected.

Very important in activating and enhancing the specific energy of the vessel.

END POINT

They are all located on the head, in particular on the face (around the eyes, sense organs).

It is very important to treat these points in the closing phase of a session, so as to converge the energies activated in the area of the forehead and eyes, which concern the connection between the brain (understand, knowing) and the ability to see life and the world.

RELEASE POINT

To stimulate the energy of the channel when you feel that it is blocked due to traumatic, emotional or climatic factors.

DIFFERENT FUNCTIONS

1 CREATION

- Origin of life.

- Continued 'recreation'.

2 CONTROL AND RESERVE

- Support of Yuan Qi for major deficits.

- Support in particular moments of life.

3 ADJUSTMENTS

- General rebalancing of their energy (Yuan Qi).

ACTIVATING THE FUNCTIONS

1 CREATION

Manual: Opening point + pathway of vessel with any specific points.

2 ADJUSTMENT

Manual: Opening point and Coupled point together + pathway of vessel and specific points.

3 RESERVE (DEFENCE)

Manual: Opening point + Release point + specific points of the Extraordinary vessels + Main channel linked to the disorder.

<u>CHONG MAI</u> Penetrating Vessel

SEA OF BLOOD

- Pathway between Pre-Heaven to Post-Heaven.

- The unfolding of the powerful life force that springs forth animating all matter between Heaven and Earth.

- The eruption of life originating from a union (the maternal and paternal Jing and the cosmic Qi).

- A gush of vitality from below (CV1) to above (following a deep internal path at the centre of the body).

- The first vessel to appear (where the Yuan Qi is concentrated). From this vessel the individual develops and takes shape: Blood, Organs, Viscera and all the meridians.

- It represents the deepest connection between Pre-Heaven (Kidney-Yin) and Post-Heaven (Stomach-Yang).

- Pushes for change (renews the blood) - difficulties changing jobs, conditions of life, marriage, home, city, stages of life, etc. and along with Ren Mai for frequent problems of the menstrual cycle, pregnancy, menopause, fertility, fecundity, menorrhagia, puberty, impotence, etc.

- Regulator of blood and the endocrine system, acts on the hair (alopecia, hirsutism, etc.) and on the skin (inelastic skin, seborrheic, adolescent acne, etc.).

- Balancing Yin-Yang of food (abdominal tract):

  KD11 - governs Yin transformations = food into matter (for problems related to excessive thinness).

  ST30- governs Yang transformations = food into energy (for problems related to being overweight).

- Origin of all organs and viscera.

  CHONG = tree   ZANG-FU = fruits

Chong Mai connects to all five organs (Zang) and to the Stomach.

Not only Sea of Blood but also the origin of SP and ST (Postnatal Qi) and also of Jin-Ye (Body Fluids) especially with the Ye (the more dense fluids), including the cerebrospinal fluid, and the hormonal and the enzymatic system.

<u>**JIN - YE**</u>   (Body Fluids)

JIN = more Yang, more fluid, more superficial (saliva, sweat, tears, etc.).

YE = more Yin, denser, deeper (blood, hormonal fluids, endocrinal fluids, cerebrospinal fluid etc.).

BLOOD STASIS:

If caused by transition =	WEI
If caused by trauma =	QIAO (BL1 end point of Qiao, connected to the hormonal system - pituitary gland).

SP4 + PC6:   very effective for harmonising Blood (transition phase)

SP4 + KD6:   very effective for harmonising Blood (if caused by trauma)

+ ST30 - SP12 - GB20

FOR PEOPLE WHO DO NOT LOVE THEMSELVES:

YIN QIAO -   REN MAI

Chong Mai may also be treated, but also in combination with the other two, otherwise it gives a boost which unblocks, but which, finding no outlet, can lead to greater closure.

- Chong Mai - Stomach (Sea of the 5 Zang)

  Stomach is closely related to the Blood which nourishes the five Zang (organs).

- Chong Mai meets at Yang Ming through Zong Jing ('ancestral muscle' fascia of abdominal muscles), which governs the whole system of bones and joints.

To open and <u>release tension in the abdomen </u>(also tension along the Chong Mai pathway), treats the entire neck area SMC (sterno-mastoid-cleido) – a very Yang Ming area - ST + LI.

1st BRANCH - CHONG MAI

Starts at CV2 (pubic bone) and follows the horizontal line of the Doors of the Earth, then travels from KD11 (sternum) along the Kidney channel as far as KD22, from where it spreads through all of the chest.

- Carries Blood to the Heart.
- Pelvis-diaphragm (chest) connection.

KD22　　　KD22

DOORS OF EARTH

SP12 - ST30 - KD11 - CV2 - KD11 - ST30 - SP12

This line is where woman often feel a blockage and it is manifested as Cold (in blockages higher up in the body they are manifested as Heat).

DISORDERS

- In menopause, when the body is no longer able to carry Blood upwards it then tends to carry up only Heat.
- For circulation:

  KD11 - Heng Hu - Pubic bone

  ST30 - Qi Chong - Qi Thoroughfare

  SP12 - Chong Men- Surging Gate

Disorders of the Lower and Middle Burner

- Genital, urinary, and gynaecological (Lower Burner).
- Digestive, rebellious Qi (Middle Burner).

ELEMENTS OF DIAGNOSIS

- Great tension/tightness of abdominal rectus muscles (taking into account the actual person: young, sporty, elderly, etc.):

      Low area -   Lower Burner (Kidneys and Yuan Qi)

      Central area – Middle Burner (Spleen and Blood)

      Upper area – Upper Burner (Upper branch and head)

- Condition of SP4.

- Tension along the line of Doors of the Earth.

- Comparison between ST30 - KD11.

TREATMENT:

SP4 -   CV2 - KD11 - ST30 - SP12 + pathway along the abdominal rectus muscles.

Treat the neck area (Tai Yang: ST - LI) helps to release tension in the abdominal muscles.

2nd BRANCH - CHONG MAI

From KD22 it continues along the pathway of the Kidney Channel (on either side of the sternum) and reaches CV22 and CV23 in the midline of the neck and from here it heads towards the face and the eyes (where it gives birth to Ren Mai)

- Relationship with Heart and Lung (Upper Burner).

- Chest Shu points are in the reverse order from the Back Shu points.

- Water is raised up to meet with Fire (Heart).

The Chest Shu points are also connected to the various Organs, but in the reverse order from the back Shu points.

CHEST SHU			BACK SHU
KD 27	SHU FU	Transport Mansion	Reunion of the Shu
KD 26	YU ZHONG	Lively Centre Water	BL23 - Kidney
KD 25	SHEN LANG	Spirit Storehouse Earth	BL20 - Spleen
KD 24	LING XU	Spirit Ruins Earth	BL18 - Liver
KD 23	FENG SHENG	Spirit Seal Fire	BL15 - Heart
KD 22	BU LANG	Corridor Walk Metal	BL13 - Lung

KD 27   Controls the other 5 points, it is a synthesis.

        Important point linking Kidney and Lung.

        Very beneficial when Lung Qi cannot descend to reach the Kidneys (dry cough or asthma).

- Cardiovascular problems (specifically for insufficient or lack of venous return).
- Children with congenital heart problems.
- Constitutional breathing problems.

Mainly influences the Heart and Lungs (Upper Burner).

ELEMENTS OF DIAGNOSIS

- Tension in the chest.
- Use Opening points to gauge state of vessel.

TREATMENT

SP4 + PC6 (linked to Heart and chest) + Kidney points on the chest (treating in particular those which have a connection with the interested organ).

For respiratory problems:

Coupled with SP4, LU7 (treatment of Chong Tai Yin).

For cardiovascular problems:

For insufficient venous return: SP4 - PC6 - LU7.

Varicose veins:

Spleen Channel + Chong Mai 2nd branch.

3rd BRANCH - CHONG MAI

Gives birth to the Du Mai. From the lower abdomen it passes through to the back and up along the spinal column.

<u>DISORDERS</u>

For constitutional problems of Yang deficiency:

- Down Syndrome in children.

- Mental retardation.

- Pregnant woman whose foetus shows signs of mental retardation.

- Degenerative problems of the spinal column, especially if linked to Blood (osteoporosis, bone cancer, etc.).

<u>ELEMENTS OF DIAGNOSIS</u>

Points of Du Mai.

<u>TREATMENT</u>

SP4 + SI3 + points of Du Mai.

Add GV4 (Ming Men) and GV14 (below the 7th cervical vertebra) as important points in activating the Yang.

4th BRANCH - CHONG MAI

From ST30 it travels in depth to meet up with the Stomach meridian, and then it goes down the leg as far as ST42.

Connected to the arterial circulation - stimulates the Yang (Stomach) to move in the Sea of Blood (Chong Mai), that is, it stimulates blood circulation.

<u>DISORDERS</u>

- Circulation problems in general.

- Collapse of the Yang (hypertension, aneurysms, arterial failure, circulation problems, etc.).

- Blood stasis (aneurysm).

- Hypertension (since it draws the Qi and Blood downwards).

<u>DIAGNOSIS</u>

Compare the pulses:

- ST 25   door of the abdomen (on either side of CV8).
- SP 12   femoral vein.
- ST 42   dorsalis pedis artery (instep).

They should have more or less the same pulse.

<u>TREATMENT</u>

SP4 - ST30 - ST42 - Chong Yang 'outpouring of Yang' (Yuan Source point of Stomach); (simultaneously apply long and deep pressure before treating the rest of the 4th Branch). Then LV3 (Tai Chong) - LV1 (Tai Yang – Yuan point) - SP1 (Yin Bai 'Hidden White').

5th BRANCH - CHONG MAI

From KD11 it follows the Kidney meridian to KD6 and YU QUAN* (below KD1).

*<u>YU QUAN</u>: is on the sole of the foot, along the midline, below KD1, at the beginning of the heel.

This point is treated in relation to foot deformity problems in children and adults (bunions, flat feet, hammer toes, etc).

- Connected to the venous circulation.
- Connects the energies of Kidney and Chong Mai (Ancestral energy par excellence).
- Gives birth to Qiao Mai.

<u>DISORDERS</u>

- Constitutional problems related to Kidneys (bone, postural, sexual, etc.).
- Foot deformity problems (hammer toes, bunions, flat feet, etc.).

<u>DIAGNOSIS</u>

- Points KD11 - KD1 - YU QUAN.

- Foot deformities (bunions, hammertoes, flat feet, etc.).

<u>TREATMENT</u>

SP4 - KD6 - KD11 (Start point) along the Kidney channel until YU QUAN.

SHU POINTS OF CHONG MAI

To treat disorders of Chong Mai.

UPPER SHU	BL 11	- intersection point of GV and CV - (Hui) Meeting point of bones
LOWER SHU	ST 37	- lower He point of LI (which along with ST constitutes Yang Ming; level of absorption, transformation and elimination).

CHONG MAI CONSTITUTION

The changes are mainly due to a Deficiency.

<u>PHYSICAL</u>

- Prevalence of the pelvis over the chest (especially the buttocks and legs). Stocky build and lover of food.

- Skin disorders (seborrheic/greasy skin, dilated skin pores, shiny complexion, adolescent acne, cellulite on hips, cold feet).

- Abundant hair.

- Prone to frequent backache, such as lumbago (rigid against change).

<u>PSYCHIC</u>

- Difficulty in making changes (everyday habits and ways of life, roles, also in the positive sense, marriage, home, work, ideas, stages of life, etc.).

- Mental rigidity, fixation.

- Feeling old before your time.

<u>SUMMARY OF THE 5 BRANCHES OF CHONG MAI</u>

1ˢᵗ BRANCH — - Gives birth to Ren Mai, to the Stomach and Kidney meridians.

- Connection between Pre-Heaven and Post-Heaven

2nd BRANCH — - Connects Water and Fire
- Carries Blood to the Heart

3rd BRANCH — - Gives birth to the Du Mai (Yang)

4th and 5th BRANCHES - Connection with Stomach and Kidney

<u>Chong Mai and erection</u>

LIVER	Yang	movement - erection
	Yin	blood - corpora cavernosa
CHONG MAI	Yang	power that bursts forth
	Yin	Sea of Blood that nourishes member

<u>For Impotence:</u>

SP4 - Stomach - CV3

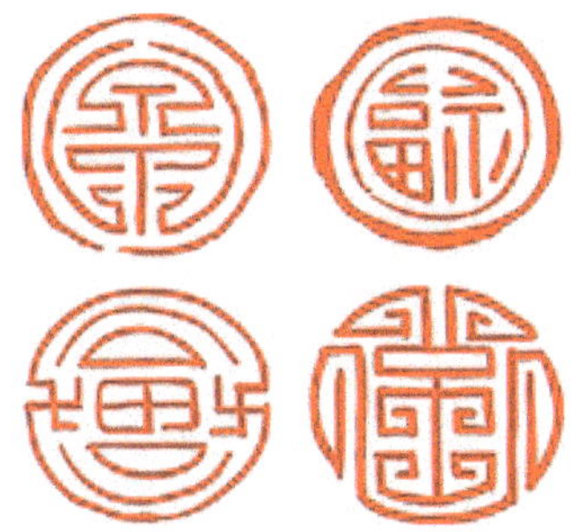

SPECIFIC POINTS OF CHONG MAI

SP 4   **Gong Sun - Grandfather Grandson**

Luo point.

- Linked to the nutrition that comes from the ancestors (maternal grandfather).
- Linked to the pelvis and reproduction; for uro-genital problems.
- Digestion (abdominal branch of the Spleen: SP12 -SP13 -SP15 -SP16).

ST 30   **Qi Chong - Qi Assault**

1 - Circulation of Qi of the abdomen:

Lower Burner

- Retention of urine and faeces
- Prolapse of the rectum
- Heat in the LI

Middle Burner

- Cold abdomen
- Abdominal pain
- Poor metabolism

UTERUS AND GENITALS

- Swelling and pain in the penis and vagina

- Retractile testicle

- Impotence / infertility

- Menstrual disorders

- Amenorrhea

- Breast-feeding difficulties

- Metrorrhagia (uterine bleeding at irregular intervals)

- Excessive menstrual flow

2 – Upper Point "Sea of Food" to restore metabolic balance.
   Yin-Yang balance with KD11.

3 - Point for "Running piglet" disorder (see Bao Mai).

KD 11   Heng Gu - Pubic Bone

Linked to Kidney and sexuality:

- Seminal losses

- Impotence / infertility

- Prolapse of the uterus and rectum

- Urinary disorders

Linked to the assimilation of food (converts food into matter).

SP 12   Chong Men - Surging Gate

- Yin Wei point (abdominal pathway).

- Moves Qi in the abdomen, especially in cases of cold.

- Point to harmonize arterio-venous flow (with ST30).

- For blood intoxication (poisoning, etc.).

- Yuan Source point (goes to the source of energy of the Stomach to enhance it and draw from it).
- Where the Chong Mai draws on the Yang:

    - arterial circulation

    - distribution of blood to the four limbs (periphery)

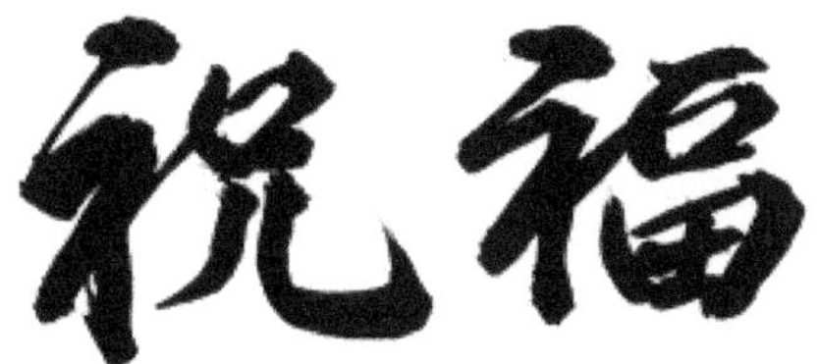

<u>REN MAI</u>   Conception Vessel

SEA OF YIN

- Taking responsibility for one's life and knowing how to nurture and preserve it.
- Loving and taking care of oneself.
- Good handling of small concrete things.
- Fostering the development of the inner self.
- Conceiving, nurturing, protecting, regulating, ordering.
- Reunion of Heaven with Earth (together with Du Mai); the Chakra are found along their pathway.
- Governs the development of the ventral and caudal parts of the foetus.

NUTRITION (together with Chong Mai)

- Menstruation
- Pregnancy
- Menopause

GROUNDING

- Solid foundation for spiritual development.

- Calms the Shen (give a concrete base and support).

- Aids the descent of the Yang (from GV20 - Hundred Meetings) so that it can join the Yin (and push the Yin upwards).

<u>YANG BLOCKED IN UPPER REGION</u>

- Hypertension.

- Hyperthyroidism (weight loss, dry and nervous gestures, emotional eating, palpitations, sweating frequent hot, flushed complexion, etc.).

- Agitation and restlessness.

- Disorders of the Shen (surrealism, eradication from the world, loss of perception of reality, alienation, mystical escapes, etc.).

- Agitated insomnia.

<u>Ren Mai pathway:</u>

Starts at CV1 (at the centre of the perineum) and goes up the anterior midline (abdomen, chest, neck, chin) until CV24 (below the lower lip); from here it splits into two branches which rise laterally to below the eyes.

<u>LUO CHANNEL OF THE REN MAI</u>

The function of the Luo Channel is to connect the depth, the level of the Blood (where the Shen resides), by bringing its energy to the brain, where all of the Longitudinal Luo meet.

They represent the link that favours change.

The Luo of Ren Mai connects and harmonizes all the Yang (Du Mai - GV1) with the Yin (Ren Mai - CV15).

Through these Luo a contact is established between the constitutional energy (8 Extraordinary Vessels) and postnatal energy (12 Main Channels).

Pathway:

GV1 - - - CV15 connection between the back and front through the psoas;

CV15 - - - GV9 connection between the front and back through the diaphragm.

Their treatment, at times, can be very effective to remove deep energetic, physical and mental blocks.

CV15   Jiu Wei – Turtle Dove Tail

- Point where the energy of Ren Mai spreads throughout the abdomen.

- Luo point of Ren Mai.

- Start point of the Divergent channel of Ren Mai.

- Being a Luo point, it activates the connection between internal and external, Yin-Yang, between Du Mai and Ren Mai and also with the Blood (which carries the Shen to the Heart).

- It is closely linked to mental rigidity:

  - tendency to repeat patterns of thought or learned behaviour (person who always shouts because he was shouted at, etc.);

  - finds it difficult to change;

  - psychosis or neurosis.

<u>REN MAI CONSTITUTION</u>

<u>PHYSICAL</u>
- Well-grounded people.
- Slightly bent forward.
- Robust and full abdomen.
- Hands slightly bent.
- Intelligent look, Yin, that penetrates deep inside.

<u>Dysfunctions</u>
- Tendency to lean forward.
- Weak back muscles and contracted abdominal muscles.
- Tendency to have a prominent abdomen.
- Kyphosis and hernias (as in a loss of shape).
- Menstrual and gynaecological disorders (as it is linked to conception).

<u>PSYCHIC</u>

- Ability to manage the material things of life and everyday pleasures.
- Introspective and intuitive capacity.
- Ability to relate to the world.
- Ability to organize.
- Take care of oneself, to love oneself.

<u>Deficit disorders</u>

- Not caring for oneself, not loving oneself.
- Lack of concreteness, making a mountain out of a molehill.
- Inconclusiveness, disorganization.
- Not standing on one's own feet (excessive dependence on others, 'psychological vampires').
- Complaining about one's fate, never satisfied.
- Not taking responsibility for one's own life.
- Inferiority complex.

<u>Excess Disorders</u>

- Obsessive care of oneself (hygienists, narcissists, excessive attention to detail, etc.).
- The need to appear, and so to flatter in order to draw attention.

Because Ren Mai and Du Mai are closely related, often a disorder in one meridian is reflected in the other.

DISORDERS AFFECTING THE THREE BURNERS:

Closely related to the entire **reproductive system** particularly for women:

- Problems related to menstruation
- Fertility
- Menopause
- Pregnancy and childbirth

<u>**Nourishes and consolidates all the Yin**</u> of the body.

- Yin Deficiency (night sweats, hot flushes, mental irritation, agitation caused by Yin deficiency, dry mouth, insomnia)

<u>**Specific action on the Uterus and Blood**</u> :

- Disorders of the menstrual cycle

- Infertility

- Menopause

- Fibroids

- Tumours

- Hernias

<u>**Facilitates the descent of Lung Qi to the Kidneys**</u> :

- Chronic asthma caused by Kidney deficiency

- Circulation of Qi in the chest (chest tightness, rapid heartbeat, anxiety)

<u>**Linked with Yuan Qi and Jing**</u> (as are all Extraordinary Vessels):

- Sexual dysfunction (impotence, sterility, etc.)

- Yin and Yang deficiency (link with Kidney, origin of Yin and Yang)

- Recovery from physical and mental exhaustion (long illness, trauma and shock, excessive work or physical activity)

<u>**Food and digestive problems**</u> :

- Form (obesity or excessive thinness) with ST30 and SP12

- Digestive difficulties (CV12 Meeting point of the six Fu organs – Mu point of ST)

- Diarrhoea

- Colic

- Lack of milk in the new mother (CV17 – on the sternum at the level of the nipples)

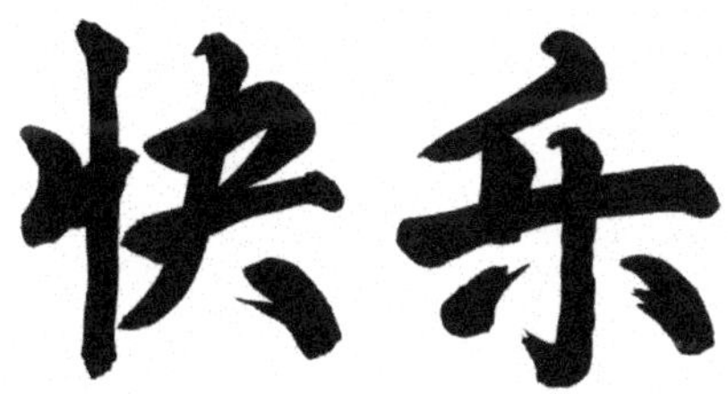

SPECIFIC POINTS OF THE CONCEPTION VESSEL (REN MAI)

CV 1   **Hui Yin – Yin Meeting Place**

Located in the centre of the perineum. It is the Start point of the Ren Mai.

Intersection point of Conception Vessel (Ren Mai), the Governing Vessel (Du Mai) and theThoroughfare Vessel (Chong Mai).

Luo point of Ren Mai.

- It has a very powerful action.
- Associated with Kidney and Uterus.
- Important point for resuscitation.
- Nourishes the Yin and the Kidney Jing (enuresis, incontinence, nocturnal emissions, etc.).
- Acts globally. Generally considered very effective in activating energy in the Extraordinary Vessels.
- Dissolves Damp-Heat in Lower Burner (genital itching, vaginal discharge, etc.).

Due to its location, CV1 can also be treated by using BL35 (Meeting of Yang) (lateral to the coccyx) with pressure towards the centre. (this point collects all the energy of CV1 and GV1 to send it upwards).

CV 2   **Qu Gù – Curved Bone**

Intersection point for lower body energy.

Point of Chong Mai.

Intersection point of Lower Yin Tendino-Muscular channel.

Intersection point of main Liver channel.

Point on Tendino-Muscular channel of the Stomach.

Divergent point with Liver and Gall Bladder.

Closely related to the genitals and fertility:

- Urinary disorders.
- Gynaecological disorders.
- Vaginal and seminal disorders.
- Andrological disorders.
- Enuresis.
- Incontinence.

CV 3   Zhong Ji – Central Pole

Point of polarity, alternating Yin and Yang.

Mu point of the Bladder.

Intersection point of the lower Yin Tendino-Muscular channel.

Intersection point of the Conception Vessel with the main channels of Spleen, Liver and Kidney.

- Urinary problems caused by Deficiency (tonifies the Bladder and stimulates the function of transformation of Qi) and by Excess (Heat-Damp).
- Problems caused by Yin deficiency (fatigue, night sweats, tired legs, lack of vitality, etc.).

CV 4   Guan Yuan – Pass Head

Supports the Kidneys, fortifies the congenital Qi (Pre-Heaven)

Mu point of Small Intestine.

Intersection point with the meridians of Spleen, Liver and Kidneys.

- One of the most important points to tonify the Qi and Blood.
- Acts on the uterus and regulates the menstrual cycle (amenorrhea, scanty periods, etc.).
- Tonifies the Kidneys and activates the Yuan Qi (chronic illnesses, weak constitution, poor state of health, etc.).
- Impotence, sterility.
- Diarrhoea (Yin deficit).
- Nourishes Xue (Blood).
- Tonifies the Yin and the Jing.
- Stabilizes the Shen caused by Empty-Heat.
- Strengthens the Qi and directs it downwards to the Lower Burner (calming effect).
- Helps the Hun to take root (nightmares).

CV 5   Shi Men – Stone Gate

Mu point of the Triple Burner.

- Spreads the Yuan Qi towards the Yin and Yang organs and towards Back Shu points.
- Moves liquids:

        - water retention

        - abdominal oedema

        - urinary retention

<u>Example:</u>   <u>Disorders of the Spleen</u>

- digestive difficulties

- loose stools

- diarrhoea

- bloating

- abdominal oedema

<u>Treatment:</u>

1 - CV5 (to move the Yuan Qi and to eliminate stagnation of fluids).

2 - Shu point of Spleen (BL20).

Mu point of Spleen (LV13)

Spleen Yuan Source point (SP3)

If necessary, you can also treat the meridian instead of just the individual points.

CV 6   Qi Hai – Sea of Qi

- Tonifies and regulates the Qi of the whole body, removes stasis.
- Invigorates the Yuan Qi and Kidney Yang (with moxa) and aids the descent the Qi into the abdomen.
- Moves Blood in the abdomen.
- Consolidates Qi in cases of exhaustion.
- Associated with the diaphragm.
- Urinary retention, oedema of the lower body (moves the Qi).
- Very effective point in cases of great physical and mental exhaustion.

CV 7   Yin Jiao – Yin Intersection

- Nourishes the Blood and Yin.
- Regulates the uterus (menstrual disorders: amenorrhea, scanty menstruation, infertility, menopause, etc.).

CV 8   Shen Qué – Spirit Gate Tower

Vigorously invigorates the Yang.

Generally this point is not treated directly but moxibustion can be used (see below).

The navel is also the memory of union, the union with the mother.

Lynch pin between Heaven and Earth:

GB26 - SP15 -ST25 - KD16 – **CV8 –** KD16 - ST25 - SP15 - GB26

The navel is very important because it is from here that the foetus obtains nourishment.

After birth nourishment is taken via the mouth (ST-SP) and nose (LU) which is again pushed down to the abdomen, the navel, where a vortex of energy is created.

It is a very sensitive area where traumas can remain registered, and therefore it is very beneficial to treat this area (area surrounding the navel).

It can be treated with moxibustion, after filling the navel with salt (severe diarrhoea), otherwise you can treat the surrounding points (KD16-ST25-VC7-VC6-VC9-VC10).

CV 9   Shui Fen – Water Divide

- Important point to regulate fluids in the body and stabilises water metabolism (transport, transformation and expulsion).

- Eliminates oedema, Dampness, Phlegm.

CV10	**CV12**	**CV13**
(Xia Wan)	**(Zhong Wan)**	**(Shan Wan)**
Lower Stomach Duct	Central Stomach Duct	Upper Stomach Duct

Linked with the Stomach (each one acts on the corresponding part of the epigastrium).

CV 10   Xia Wan - Lower Stomach Duct

Intersection point with the Spleen and Small Intestine channels

- Aids digestion (eliminates food stagnation, stimulates circulation of Stomach Qi).
- Acts on ST and SP.
- Abdominal distention, bloating, feeling of fullness, etc.

CV 11   Jian Li – Iinterior Strengthening

- Stimulates the descent of Stomach Qi.
- Aids digestion (feeling of fullness and bloating, nausea, vomiting, pain, etc.).
- More effective in syndromes of Excess.

CV 12   Zhong Wan – Central Stomach Duct

Mu point of the Stomach and Middle Burner.
Meeting (Hui) point for the six Fu organs.

- Invigorates the Qi of Stomach and Spleen.
- Dissolves Phlegm and Dampness.
- Governs all digestive functions.
- Acts globally on all digestive processes, but is more effective in Deficit syndromes.
- Inability to "digest" life.
- Heartburn, ulcers.

CV 13   Shang Wan – Upper Stomach Duct

- Subdues rebellious Stomach Qi (belching, nausea, vomiting, hiccups, sense of fullness, etc.).
- Connects Stomach to Heart.
- More effective in syndromes of Excess.

CV 14   Ju Qué - Great Tower Gate

Mu point of the Heart.

- Strong association with the diaphragm.
- "Leads to the heart."
- Digestive problems linked to emotional disorders.
- Tonifies and regulates Heart, Spleen, Lung and Stomach Qi.
- Relaxes the abdomen.
- Calms the Shen.
- Invigorates Heart Blood.

CV 15   Jiu Wei – Turtledove Tail

Luo point of the Conception Vessel (Ren Mai).

(Yuan) Source point of 5 Yin Organs.

- From this point the energy of the Ren Mai spreads throughout the abdomen.
- For mental rigidity.
- Invigorates Heart Blood.
- Calms the Shen (especially in cases of restlessness, severe anxiety, worry, fear, obsessions, etc.).
- Nourishes all the organs.

CV 17   Dan Zhong – Chest Centre

Mu point of Pericardium.

Mu point of the Upper Burner.

(Hui) Meeting point of the Qi.

Sea of Qi point.

- Regulates the Qi and Blood in the chest and stimulates the circulation of Zong Qi.
- Stimulates Defensive Qi (Wei Qi).
- 'Opening up to the world'.
- Stimulates descent of rebellious Qi (Ni Qi).
- Benefits breastfeeding.
- Invigorates the Qi of the Upper Burner and dispels stasis (tightness in the chest, shortness of breath, chest pain, etc.).

- Tonifies and regulates Lung Qi (cough and chronic bronchitis, asthma, shortness of breath, sadness, etc.).
- For everything linked to Heart (heart pain, sadness, etc.).
- Hiatal hernia.

CV 22   Tian You – Celestial Chimney

Yin Wei Mai and Chong Mai point.

Window of the Sky point.

- Stimulates the descent of Lung Qi (asthma, acute and chronic cough, dry mouth, loss of voice, globus hystericus (sensation of a lump in the throat), thyroid disease, etc.).
- Dispels Phlegm in the Lungs and throat and promotes expectoration of phlegm.
- Clears Lung Heat.

CV 23   Lian Quan – Ridge Spring

Yin Wei Mai point (Yin Linking Vessel).

- Stimulates the function of speech, especially after a Cerebro-Vascular attack.
- Dispels internal Wind and Phlegm.
- Purifies Fire.
- Subdues rebellious Qi.

CV 24   Cheng Jiang – Sauce Receptacle

- Disperse external Wind (facial paralysis).

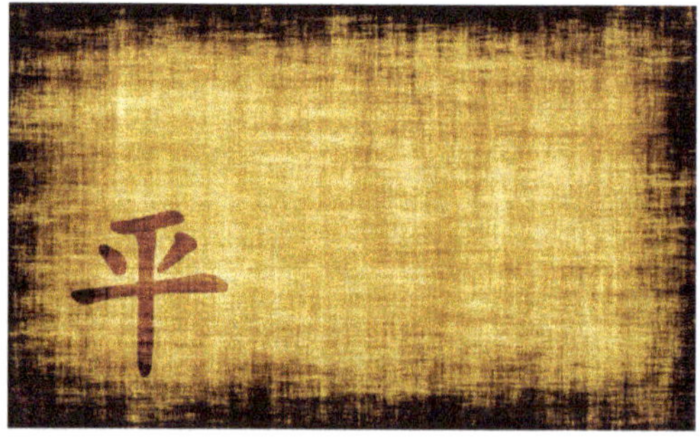

<u>DU MAI</u>   Governing Vessel

SEA OF YANG

"Growth controller by hand and eye."
The ability to stand erect, thanks to a vital upward thrust, to fulfil one's destiny.

- The father who governs and controls the development of the child, so that it is ordered, harmonious and have a clear direction.

- Set goals and pursue them.

- Foster the development of potential through solid intent and clear determination.

- Governs the development of the dorsal and cranial areas in the foetus.

- Tonifies all Yang.

- Strengthens the spine.

- Nourishes the Marrow and Brain, supplying it with the Kidney Jing.

- Dispels external Wind (headache, fever, runny nose, etc.) and internal Wind (dizziness, seizures, tremors, seizures, etc.).
  (Wind symbolically indicates change).

- Encapsulates the functions of the Zang-Fu but at a deeper level. In fact, the points on the Governing Vessel affect the organ belonging to the Shu point located at the same level on the back.

- Distributes, circulates, connects (Yang functions).

<u>Pathway of the Governing Vessel (Du Mai):</u>

From GV1 (midway between the tip of coccyx and the anus) it goes up along the centre of the spine, to the top of the head, to then go downwards again towards the forehead, and nose and ending at GV28, on the inside of the upper lip (junction between gum and upper lip).

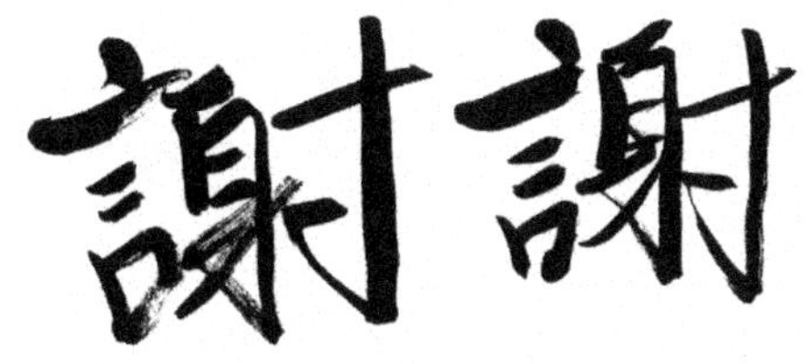

MEETING POINTS

Points that connect with different Main Channels.

GV 1 -   Ren Mai / Kidney / GB

GV 13 -   Bladder

GV 14 -   all 6 Yang Channels

GV 15 -   Yang Wei

GV 17 -   Bladder

GV 20 -   All the Yang

GV 24 -   Bladder / Stomach

GV 26 -   LI / Stomach

GV 28 -   Ren Mai / Stomach

LUO CHANNEL OF DU MAI

Originates at GV1 (midway between tip of coccyx and the anus), goes up either side of the spine to the height of GV12, where it makes contact with BL12 where it then goes to GV13 (forming a sort of rhombus called 'The Diamond'); from this point it continues upwards on either side of spine to GV16 (base of the neck) where it then descends to the area of the Kidneys.

- Stiffness along the spinal column (excess in the Luo Du Mai).

- Heaviness of the head (which tends to nod) - (Deficit problem).

- Spinal cord injury.

Treat: GV1 (Luo Du Mai) + Luo points (on either side of spinal column) + GV12 (parallel to BL13 - Shu point of the Lung) + BL35

GV 14   **Yang (of the Heart)**   to sedate the Yang

GV 4   **Yang (of the Kidney)** to tonifiy the Yang

<u>THE DIAMOND:</u>   GV 12 – BL 12 - GV 13

This area effectively activates the Luo Du Mai.

Linked to the distribution of Qi (BL12 above BL13 Shu point of Lung) and linked to
    Wind (BL11 -BL12), and as such, it facilitates movement and change.

The Luo Du Mai, in particular, brings Du Mai energy to the brain (treats cases of spinal
cord injury that have caused a paraplegia).

Luo Du Mai (GV 1) + Yang Qiao points (for unresolved physical or mental trauma) +
GB39 (Meeting point of the Bone Marrow) + BL11 (Meeting point of the bones).

<u>1st SECONDARY BRANCH - DU MAI</u>

It starts at CV2, passes deep within the abdomen, up through the navel, and then up to the
Heart, throat and face, finishing at BL1.

- Lower abdominal pain that extends upwards towards the heart.

- Haemorrhoids.

- Urinary incontinence.

- Infertility.

<u>Specific treatment:</u>   CV 2 coupled with local points.

<u>2nd SECONDARY BRANCH - DU MAI</u>

From CV2 it goes up along the sides of the spinal column as far as BL1, where it enters the
brain and, always via the Bladder Meridian, it travels down to BL23, where it enters the
Kidneys.

- Contractures of the back and neck.

- Sensation of energy rising upwards.

- Pain in the hips.

- Headache.

- Sub-orbital neuralgia.

<u>Specific treatment:</u>   CV 2 and local points.

GV 4 - when excessive physical activity has caused rigidity in lumbar region.

GV 14 - when excessive mental activity has caused rigidity in the cervical region.

SEPARATION OF THE CHILD FROM THE MOTHER

The Governing Vessel (Du Mai) provides the impetus that allows the child to become independent and separate itself from the mother.

- weaning

- standing upright to walk

- teething

- talking

<u>Excessive attachment:</u> Yang deficiency (lack of autonomy).

<u>Premature separation:</u> Excess of Yang (restless sleep, irritability, agitation, tremors, etc).

DU MAI CONSTITUTION

PHYSICAL

- Tall people (or perceived to be tall).
- Paravertebral muscles well developed.
- Posture with open shoulders.
- Bright, magnetic look, looks ahead.

<u>Disorders:</u>

- Hypertrophy or strong contractions of the paravertebral muscles.
- Stiffness of the trunk.
- Expansion or contraction of the chest.
- Scoliosis.
- Central or bilateral backache (never unilateral).
- Lower back pain, finds it difficult to lie flat.

<u>PSYCHIC</u>

- Charismatic individuals, with strong personalities, tending to control, organize, direct.
- People able to conceive and carry out grand projects, to achieve great goals.
- Ability to recreate themselves and to move forward even in the face of adversity.
- Tendency to perfectionism and efficiency.
- Logical and rational.

<u>Disorders:</u>
- Megalomania and tendency to overwhelm.
- Sense of omnipotence.
- Lack of awareness of limits.
- Excessive mental activity.
- Tendency to be perpetually dissatisfied.

<u>SIGNS AND SYMPTOMS</u>

- Rigidity of the spine.
- Internal Wind: (restlessness, agitation, madness, tremors, convulsions, epilepsy, etc.).
- External Wind: (GV14 Great Hammer / 7th cervical vertebra) - (severe headache, high fever, runny nose, etc.).
- Yang Deficiency: (GV4 - Ming Men) - (lumbar pain, cold hands and knees, fatigue, sluggish digestion, etc.).
- Excess of Yang: (GV14 Great Hammer / 7th cervical vertebra) - (stiffness and pain in the shoulders and neck 'Bison's hump').
- Jing does not reach the brain (amnesia, confusion, difficulty concentrating, mental retardation, etc.).

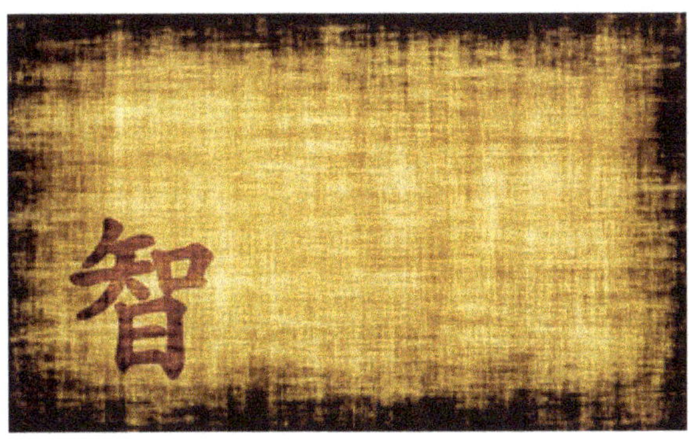

The curvatures of the spinal column create three great centres (pelvis, chest, brain) that correspond to the three levels of energy (Jing, Qi, Shen):

Brain	BL1 / GV20	Adult	EVOLUTION
SHEN			Awareness of others
Chest	GV9	Adolescence	INTERRELATION
QI			"I with others" the social being (includes feelings)
Pelvis	GV1	Childhood	SURVIVAL
JING		Birth	"I"

GENERAL FUNCTIONS OF DU MAI

- Tonifies the Yang (especially Kidney Yang)
- Dispels the Wind (internal and external)
- Strengthens the spinal column
- Nourish the marrow and the brain

SPECIFIC POINTS OF THE GOVERNING VESSEL (DU MAI)

GV 1   Chang Qiang - Long Strong

Luo point of GV.

- Removes obstructions from GV and CV.
- Supports growth.
- Strengthens the spinal column.
- Local point for prolapse of the anus.
- Expels Damp-Heat from the anus (haemorrhoids).
- Calms the Shen.
- Acts on the highest region (brain).

<u>SYMPTOMS:</u>

1 - Lower Burner:

- Prolapsed uterus or anus

- Haemorrhoids

- Genital disorders

- Premature Ejaculation

- Coccyx pain

- Etc.

2 - Yang:

- Rigidity of the spinal column

- Convulsions

3 - Deficit of Yang in the upper region:

- Heavy head

- Fuddled mind

GV 2   Yao Shu - Lumbar Transport

- Tonifies the lower back.
- Tonifies the Kidneys.
- Tonifies the legs (for Bi syndromes)
- Eliminates internal Wind (epilepsy, spasms, convulsions, etc.).

GV 3   Yao Yang Guan - Lumbar Yang Pass

- Very useful for lumbar hernias (between L4 and L5).
- Tonifies lower back and limbs.
- Strengthens the legs and knees (considered an extension of Kidneys to which the knees are energetically related - cold knees = Kidney Deficit).
- Intestinal disorders (associated with Shu point of LI -BL25).

GV 4   **Ming Men - Life Gate (name often used to describe all of this area)**

- Great point for tonification of the Yang in general and of the Kidney Yang.
- Strengthens the Fire of Ming Men (which in turn facilitates the transformation of Water).
- This point should always be tonified, never sedated, but if anything, the Qi can be directed elsewhere.
- Strengthens the Yuan Qi (chronic physical and mental weakness, fatigue, etc.).
- Expels internal Cold.
- Strengthens the lower back and knees.
- High fever.
- Nourishes the Jing (frigidity, impotence, premature ejaculation, etc.).
- Nourishes the Blood.
- Tonifies the Liver.
- Expels Wind.
- Irregular menstruation.
- Haemorrhoids.
- Loss of liquids in lower part of body (diarrhoea, leucorrhoea, spermatorrhea, enuresis, etc.).

GV 6   **Ji Zhong - Spinal Centre**

Lies below the spinous process of the 11th thoracic vertebra.

At the side of Shu point of Spleen (BL20).

- To treat Middle Burner: SP + ST (Fire).

GV 7   **Zhong Shu - Central Pivot**

Lies below 10th thoracic vertebra

Beside Shu point of GB (BL19).

- To treat GB as an Extraordinary Fu Viscera.

GV 8   **Jin Suo - Sinew Contraction**

- Muscle spasms (related to Liver).
- Muscle atrophy (e.g after a long illness).
- Anger, agitation.
- Problems related to Parkinson's disease.

GV 9   Zhi Yang - Extremity of Yang

It lies at the end of the dorsal curvature (7th – 8th thoracic vertebra).

- Disorders of the Upper Burner (HT + LU).
- Mobilizes the Qi in the Middle Burner.
- Treats problems or blockages in the diaphragm (breathing, digestion, etc.).
- Regulates LV and GB.
- Drains Damp-Heat in the chest, in the GB and LV.

Example: Blockages at the level of the diaphragm

       <u>QI</u>
- Agitation
- Shortness of breath
- Palpitations
- Anxieties
- Restlessness, etc.

       <u>BLOOD</u>
- Blocked menstrual cycle
- Circulatory problems
- Hypertension

Treatment:

CV 15	Removes stiffness
GV 1	(BL35) Luo point of GV
SP 21	Great point for freeing up the chest, for severe pain
GV 9	For blockages in the diaphragm
BL 17	Shu point of the diaphragm (at the side of GV9)
CV 17	For everything concerning LU and HT, 'open up to the world'
GB 25	'Jing Men' for tensions in the chest, makes Qi flow in Lower Burner
HT 1	Highest Spring (Ji Quan)

GV 10   Ling Tai - Spirit Tower

Lies just below Du Shu (Shu point of Du Mai) BL16 (6th thoracic vertebra).

- Acts on the Du Mai.

GV 11   Shen Dao - Spirit Path

Lies on same level as Shu point of the Heart (BL15) - 5th thoracic vertebra.

- Calms the Shen.

- Regulates the Heart (agitation, tachycardia, etc.).

GV 12   Shen Zhu - Body Pillar

- Eliminates internal Wind (spasms, convulsions, tremors, epilepsy, etc.).
- Tonifies the Lungs.
- Strengthens the body after a long illness.

GV 13   Tao Dao - Kiln Path

Meeting point with the Bladder meridian.

- Shapes our path, creates, shapes who we are.
- Purifies the Heat, especially Heat of the Heart.
- Point known by the name "hundred fatigues".

GV 14   Da Zhui - Great Hammer

In the depression below the spinous process of the 7th cervical vertebra.

Meeting point with the meridians of BL, GB, and ST.

Intersection point linking with all six Yang channels.

- Disperses excess Heat (fever, hypertension, "bison's hump", etc.).
- Disperses Dampness.
- Purifies Fire.
- Acts on Heart Yang.
- Stimulates the Marrow to reach the brain.

GV 16   Feng Fu - Wind Mansion

Point of Yang Wei Mai.

Point of Sea Marrow.

- Expels internal and external Wind.
- Frees the head.
- Brings the pure essence to the brain.

GV 17   Nao Hù - Brain's Door

Intersection point with Bladder meridian.

- Eliminates internal Wind.
- Brings clarity to the brain (disorientation).
- Neuralgia, occipital headache.

GV 19   Hou Ding - Behind the Vertex

- Strong calming effect on the Shen (coupled with CV15).

GV 20   Bai Hui - Hundred Convergences

Intersection point with all the Yang channels.

Sea Marrow point.

- Raises Yang to the head and purifies the mind.
- Related to prolapse (uterus, stomach, bladder, anus, vagina).
- Resuscitation point (restores the state of consciousness).
- Subdues internal Wind.
- Depression, low spirits, etc.
- High or low pressure.
- Haemorrhoids.
- Poor memory.
- Enables Marrow to fill the brain.

GV 23   Shang Xing - Upper Star

- Star that gives direction, directs the Shen (bright temple).
- Disorientation, confusion.
- Acts on the nose (chronic problems of sinusitis, allergic rhinitis, nasal congestion, etc.).
- Dissolves Phlegm.

GV 24   Shen Ting - Spirit Court

Intersection point with Stomach meridian.

- Very effective in calming the Shen (severe anxiety, fear, schizophrenia, etc.).
- Regulates the Heart (agitation, tachycardia, etc.).

GV 26   Ren Zhong/Shui Gou - Water Trough

- Restores contact between Earth (mouth) and Heaven (nose).
- Point of resuscitation.
- For lockjaw (clenched jaw due to spasmodic contraction of the masseter).
- Bruxism.
- Lumbago.
- Strong action on the pelvis.
- Urinary problems caused by spasms.
- Restores consciousness after epileptic seizures.

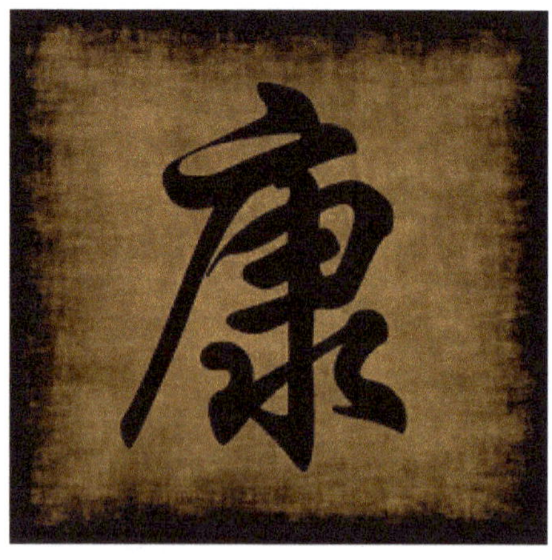

<u>DAI MAI</u>   Girdling Vessel

A belt that encircles and wraps round us to give us:

- Cohesion

- Solidity

- Stability

- Balance

- Containment

- Circulation

- Protection

- Contemplation

- Support

- Union

- Order

- The Girdling Vessel (Dai Mai) encircles the body like a belt and thus connects with all the Main and Extraordinary channels and is connected to all the Zang-Fu (through its function to connect and circulate).

- The area where the original Essence (Dan Dien and Ming Men) resides.

- Connection with Zong Jin (Ancestral muscle).

- Tightly bound to GB (or, rather, vice versa) for judgment and decision.

- Strongly linked to Post-Heaven and therefore to the energy that we take from the outside world.

- Ability to digest and dispose of what is no longer of use, to eliminate, to free oneself of unnecessary accumulations that create stagnation, especially in the Lower Burner.

(In the case of the LI, holding on, not being unable to let go is associated with the present, everyday situations, whereas in the Dai Mai, it is another type of retention, a long term inability to let go; a hoarding of obsolete things over time, of things that are no longer of any use, and also of sentiments like resentment and jealousy.)

<u>The Pathway of the Girdling Vessel - Dai Mai</u>:

Starts at CV1, continues to GV4 and then extends to the sides, passing through LV13, GB26, GB27 and GB28, to finally reach CV8.

DAI MAI CONSTITUTION

<u>PHYSICAL</u>

- Strength, vigour and cohesion.

- Upper body strong and hot and the lower body solid and stable.

- Waist area elastic and toned.

<u>Disorders</u>

- Pear shaped body, narrow at the top and obese lower down. Upper part excessively strong and hot (especially the hands) and the lower part cold (with cellulite).
The Yang that stays in the upper region will lead to excessive tension and contraction of the neck muscles while the part below the waist will be flaccid and spreading.
Feeling as if divided in two.

- A dislike of belts or things that tighten round the waist and hips.

- Constipation or diarrhoea with unformed faeces.

- Digestive problems.

- Lower back pain.

- Leucorrhoea.

YANG IN UPPER BODY

- Hot hands

- Hot chest

- Chest tightness

- Palpitations

- Tension in neck muscles

- Agitation, restlessness

YIN IN LOWER BODY

- Cold feet

- Cellulite

- Abdominal distention

- Tumours (masses, fibroids, cysts, etc.)

- Feeling of sitting in cold water

<u>PSYCHOLOGICAL</u>

- Ability to give cohesion, unity and support.

- Coherence, both internally and externally.

- Ability to move and navigate easily and decisively, both in the outside world and in one's personal life.

- Judgment and decision (linked with GB).

- Disciplined, orderly and structured.

<u>Disorders</u>

- Total disorder or obsessive neatness.

- Lost.

- Inability to move in a coherent and orderly way.

- To have no clear direction (and so unable to complete a task).

- Hypercritical.

- Intolerant.

- Discomfort at being in the world and so retreating into oneself.

Dai Mai can easily have a crisis during stages of transition in life.

<u>BLOCKAGE OF THE DAI MAI</u>

All disorders of the Dai Mai refer to accumulation which creates stagnation and can relate to the Lower, Middle and Upper Burner.

The problems of the Dai Mai do not affect the meridian directly, but can be noted elsewhere or affect a certain organ.

LOWER BURNER

<u>COLD</u>

- Abdominal masses (fibroids, cysts, tumours, etc.).

- Leucorrhoea (linked to the Kidney function, its elimination process).

- Impotence / infertility.

- Pain and cold in the lumbosacral area.

MIDDLE BURNER

DIGESTION

- Stomach - Spleen.

- Stasis and/or deficit.

(Qi deficiency can be deep rooted and hidden by surface tension and contraction of the abdominal muscles - specific point to treat: ST32).

DAMPNESS

- Due to stagnation (Cold or Hot).

Originates in the Spleen and transfers to LV13 (Mu point of Spleen) then GB26, GB27 and GB28, in an attempt to descend.
The body will try to transform it into Heat, which, by ascending, it can be expelled, if it does not succeed, there will be signs of Heat in the Upper Burner (Heart - irritability, panic attacks, anxiety, etc.).
If the Heat is unable to rise, it will give signs of Heat in the Lower Burner (inflammation of the genitals).
If Dampness remains Cold and stagnant in the Lower Burner, the signs may be: vaginal discharge, cystitis, vaginitis, urinary tract infections, diarrhoea, loose stools, impotence, infertility, fibroids, intestinal abscess; also a feeling of heaviness in the lower back and the iliac crests, lumbar pain that extends to the front (along the pathway of the Dai Mai).

UPPER BURNER

HEAT

Many psycho-behavioural signs: restlessness, agitation, anxiety, panic, etc.

Example:

Leucorrhea (white vaginal discharge) caused by Cold and Heat (yellow discharge) with disorders related to stagnation.

       Ovulation

Yin   Yang

Cold   Hot

       Menstruation

       Period of Deficit:

       - Yin (Xue)

       - Yang

- Spleen in Yin phase
- Liver in Yang phase

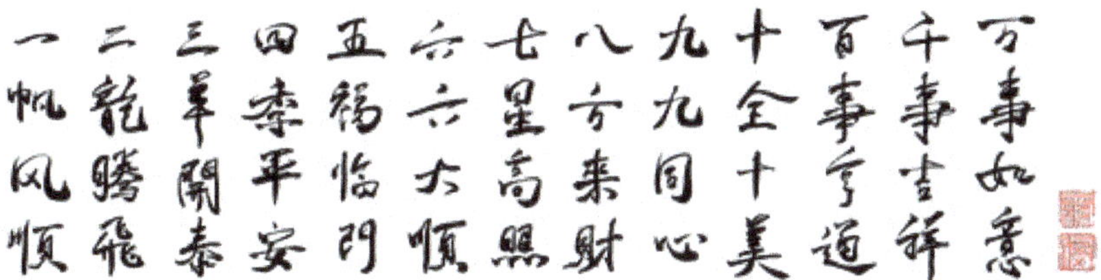

BAO MAI

The Bao Mai is an extension of the Dai Mai. It is the vessel that permits the "Pilgrimage of Water to the Heart" i.e the connection between Jing (KD) and Shen (HT).

The Water, the Jing, which resides in the Kidneys, must join the Fire of the Heart to allow the individual to grow and evolve, developing their individuality, to make experiences in life and to fulfil their own destiny (Ming Men).

This can be brought about through the Bao Mai; it is the extension of the Dai Mai and spreads its opening movement and communication.

Binds and connects the front and back and the various rings (from CV8 to GV1 it ascends along the spinal column to GV9 and then passes to the front to CV15).

Typical Disorder:

"RUNNING PIGLET DISORDER":

- Sense of movement in the abdomen that is trying to rise into the chest to escape but without success, causing a blockage at the level of the diaphragm;
- State of deep anxiety;
- Sense of constriction, but also of strong movement in the abdomen;
- Something strong that moves but gets nowhere;
- Sense of loss and mental confusion;
- Panic attacks (Upper Burner) combined with visceral anxiety (Middle and Lower Burner).

<u>TREATMENT OF DAI AND BAO MAI</u>

In all cases of stagnation, to free the Dai Mai, one should first deal with the Bao Mai, treating the area of the chest and in particular GV9 and BL17 on the back, and CV17 and CV15 on the front.

In cases of severe constriction in the abdomen, there will also be tension found in the chest; so, firstly, it is necessary to relax the chest.

If, on the other hand, there is a problem of the Bao Mai (Running Piglet Disorder) it should be treated in the reverse order (first open the Dai Mai and then treat the Bao Mai).

LV 5   Luo connecting point of Liver

GV 1   Luo connecting point of GB

CV 15   Luo connecting point of CV

SP 21   Great Luo connecting point of Spleen

GV 1   For disorders of a more Yang nature (panic attacks, anxiety, etc.)

CV 15   For disorders of a more Yin nature (cystitis, breast lumps, etc.)

Alternatively, you can use BL17 instead of GV1.

You can start by applying gentle, constant pressure on LV5 and GB41, and then proceed with the Bao Mai from the navel along the CV (Ren Mai) to CV2 and then take the GV (Du Mai) to GV9. Then Dai Mai from GV, paying particular attention to SP21, GB22 and GB23.

SPECIFIC POINTS OF THE GIRDLING VESSEL (DAI MAI)

LV 13   Zhang Men – Camphorwood Gate (completeness)

Intersection of the Dai Mai (Girdling Vessel) with Spleen (Post-Heaven).

Mu point of the Spleen.

Meeting point for all the viscera (Fu organs).

-   To digest (let go).

LV 14   Qi Men – Cycle Gate

Mu point of the Liver.

GB 26   Dai Mai – Girdling Vessel

- Encapsulates the Dai Mai.
- Effectively connects upper and lower (HT - KD).

Upper:

- Intercostal Pain
- Expanding waistline
- Oppression

Lower:

- Pain in the groin
- Inguinal hernias
- Prolapses
- Vaginal discharge

GB 27   Wu Shu – Fifth Pivot

To direct Qi down into Lower Burner.

In Men:

- Retraction of the testicle
- Back pain
- Tension, contractions, spasms, hernias, etc.

In Women:

- Prolapsed uterus
- Discharge
- Menstrual problems in general

GB 28   Wei Dao – Linking Path

Its action is very similar to GB27.

<u>DAI MAI</u>

KIDNEY: Expression of the strength of the Kidneys (associated with GV4 -BL23 Kidney Divergent).

LV and GB: Expression of movement and communication. The energy of Kidney that is set in motion (pathway with the following points LV13 and GB26, GB27, GB28).

SPLEEN: Supports, maintains shape (LV13 = Mu point of Spleen, the Middle Burner area, navel = centre).

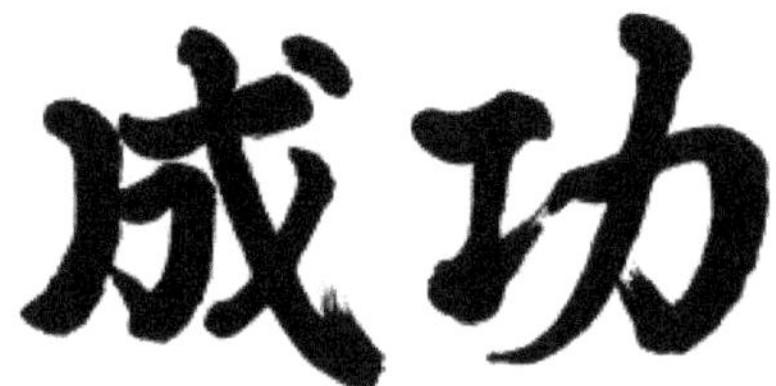

<u>REN MAI</u>	<u>DU MAI</u>	<u>CHONG MAI</u>	<u>DAI MAI</u>
CIFOSIS LORDOSIS	SCOLIOSIS	EXPANSION OF LOWER BODY	FLAT BACK
	The upward thrust is blocked by the weight of life.	Vital thrust is insufficient	<u>Deficit</u>: expanding waistline and hips
			<u>Excess</u>: narrowing of the waist and hips

<u>WEI MAI</u>   Linking Vessels

"A connection to allow flight, free movement".

- Initiative and vitality.
- Links the various stages of life (birth, childhood, adolescence, adulthood, old age, death), harmonizing the steps between them.
- Useful as a support and help in each transitional age.
- Allows movement, expression of life, giving a sense of uniqueness that is made up of moments, stages.
- Slows down the progress of degenerative factors.
- Problems related to aging.
- Linked to the 7-8 year cycle.

<u>CYCLES:</u>

Women:	7 years, odd (yang) to balance the feminine Yin.
Men:	8 years, even (yin) to balance the masculine Yang.

Each cycle represents the availability of the Yuan Qi, and therefore the Jing of each individual.

The Yuan Qi continues to be generated for 5 cycles (which correspond to the 5 elements) according to the time sequence that starts with the Wood element (Wood - Fire - Earth - Metal - Water).

When this process reaches its climax with the element Water, it starts to go backwards in the reverse order (Water - Metal - Earth - Fire - Wood) decreasing the availability of Yuan Qi for another 5 cycles until death.

The woman, who, in many ways is more related to Jing, which is Yin, tends to consume the Vital Essence more steadily (for example, through the menstrual cycle), while the man being more Yang, tends to consume the Jing more rapidly.

<u>Menopause and aging in women:</u> the symptoms are mainly connected to the decline of Yin (osteoporosis, fibroids, hormonal cycle disorders, etc.).

<u>Andropause and aging in men:</u> the symptoms are mainly connected to the decline of Yang (heart problems, decline in mental ability, impotence, etc.).

If a person nourishes and conserves his essence, he can start another cycle.

<u>Saturation points</u>

Woman 7 x 7 = 49 completion of Yin

Man   8 x 8 = 64 completion of Yang

Two important stock taking phases (what is done is done) from the physiological point of view, career, realisation, etc.

Two points of completion, from where one can also start to dedicate oneself to other things.

FUNCTIONS OF THE WEI

Follow and help man in the various transitional stages of life.

Key points to help the individual to grow during two stages of life:

GB 29   Transition point from childhood to adolescence

SI 10   Transition point to adulthood

If these points are very painful even in old age, it may indicate that there were traumas or difficulties during the related transition period.

The Wei represent the first move towards life, the transition towards living.

Related to the use of the energetic inheritance, represented by Fire (Heart: seat of Shen) and Water (Kidneys: seat of Jing).

The Heart represents experience (both the experiencing of life and learning from it), which, for it to be lived, requires Kidney energy. The action of the Heart that burns life.

From this, the bond between the Heart and the Brain (seat of experience-memory) also called 'Sea of Marrow' (union of Jing and Shen).

Marrow = also called Kidney Yang

Bone = also called Kidney Yin

At birth a connection is formed between the external Qi and the internal Qi: Lung (Metal) connects to Kidneys (Water). Through the act of taking breath, the external Qi is pushed downwards to the Kidneys.

The Lung sends Qi downwards and the Kidneys collect the Lung Qi.

The Tai Yin (Lung/Spleen - the most superficial aspect of Yin, the great Yin which goes towards the Yang) enters into contact with Shao Yin (Water - the youngest and most profound aspect, in the sense of the beginning of life) to bring it to the surface.

LU7 and SP4 (Tai Yin – superficial) are Luo connecting points and Meeting points of the Ren Mai and Chong Mai (depth – the most Yin Extraordinary vessels).

<u>Takes from the outside</u>

Air   Food and Water

LUNG   Tai Yin   SPLEEN

LU7   Luo Points   SP4

<u>Draws it deep down inside</u>

Kidneys (Shao Yin)

Yin Qiao   KD6

<u>And brings back to the surface and distributes all that was drawn deep down</u>

Heart (Shao Yin)

Yin Wei - PC6

<u>YANG WEI</u>

The Yang Wei Vessel starts at BL63, passes through GB35 and goes straight to GB29 and then up to SI10, where it branches off towards TB13, LI14, TB15, while another branch continues to GB21, GV15, GV16, GB20, GB14 to finish on the forehead (GB13 - ST8).

- The free expression of the potential of living (as you make choices, that which is potentiality becomes reality).

- The reduction in the possibility to choose comes with the consumption of life.

    Water-Fire conflict = TB (the channel that spreads the Yuan Qi, the Jing activated by the original Yang to become Qi -TB5 Opening point of Yang Wei).

- Connected to the corpus callosum connecting the two hemispheres of the brain, allowing us to translate thought into action, that is, choose and act and then consume the life.

- Connected to GB (the viscera responsible for making decisions).

- Nutrition, choice, change, transformation.

- Given that making choices implies movement/motility on all three energetic levels (Yang), this is why we find the following points along the Yang Wei Vessel: Tai Yang (BL63), Shao Yang (GB35), Tai Yang (SI10), Yang Ming (LI14) and again Shao Yang (TB13 and TB15).

BL 63   **Jin Men - Metal Gate**

(Xi) Cleft point of Bladder.

- The door through which we begin to take a look outside.
- Metal (LU) represents the opening up to life on the Water channel (Tai Yin, which, from the inside, moves to the outside - Yang).
- The Tai Yang that moves and breathes life.
- Beside BL63, BL61 'Child Gate' is located.
- To open the energy of the channel, open towards life, when a person is very indecisive and discouraged.

GB 35   **Yang Jiao - Yang Intersection**

(Xi) Cleft point of the Yang Wei.

- Opening, choose.
- Yang Intersection.
- Transition point from the Tai Yang (BL63) to the Shao Yang (GB35).

GB 29   **Ju Liao - Squatting Bone-Hole**

- Yang Wei / Yang Qiao.
- For Peter Pan syndrome.

Three levels of Yang:

SI10   Tai Yang "Adult Gate" (knowledge, act as an adult)

LI14   Yang Ming

TB 13-15   Shao Yang

<u>Energy entry points to the brain</u> (the awareness of experience gained through the choices one makes):

GB20	Feng Chi – Wind Pool
GB13	Ben Shen – Root Spirit
GB14	Yang Bai – Yang White
ST8	Tou Wei – Head Corner

BL35   Hui Yang - Meeting of Yang

Lateral to the coccyx.

- Point where all the Yang meet.
- Point that consolidates the energy of Lower Burner and then promotes its circulation. 'Consolidates the Yang in Lower Burner'.
  'Gathers' the Yang in order to take it back to the centre (GV1 Long Strong) and to the spinal column.
- Great point to act on Yang Wei even if it is not on its actual pathway.

BL 61   Child Gate

GB 29   Adolescent Gate (for Peter Pan syndromes)

SI 10   Adult Gate

GB 20   Feng Chi - Wind Pool

Wind = movement, change, choices

Pool = life experience

Point of choice making (headache = inability to choose).

Entry point to awareness born of experience.

BL 4   **Qu Cha - Deviating Turn**

Connect, referring to the brain.

- Alzheimer.

YIN WEI

Starts at KD9, goes up along the inside of the leg to SP12 and follows the points SP13, SP15, SP16 and LV14, and from here it connects to CV22 and then CV23 to finish on the face.

- It consumes life at a concrete level. Like the Yang Wei, the Yin Wei is involved in the connection and the use of Jing, but in a more material and structural way (it ensures the distribution of the Kidney Jing to the body and connects the interior with the exterior - the Yin with the Yang).
- Connected to the consumption of Jing at all stages of life, particularly in old age (the potential becomes reality).
- From Pre-Heaven (Kidneys), transports the energy to the Post-Heaven (Spleen), spreading it, involving the Liver, finally reaching the head.
- Treat the Yin Wei vessel to help a person to optimize the process of distribution and consumption of energy.

CONSUMPTION OF KIDNEY JING

To gain experience of life (Heart)

(aging)

connecting to the Post-Heaven (Spleen)

spreading the energy – Pre-Heaven and Post-Heaven (Liver)

and bringing it to the head to facilitate awareness/consciousness.

SPECIFIC POINTS OF YIN WEI

KD 9   **Zhu Bin - Guest House**

Zhu = House

Bin = Guest

(Xi) Cleft point and Start point of the Yin Wei vessel.

- The Kidneys offer to the guest (Yin Wei).
- Where construction starts.
- The point to treat if you wish to have "a son who laughs all day and sleeps all night" (point to be treated in the third, sixth and ninth month of pregnancy).
- To impede the transmission of disease from mother to child (to be treated in pregnancy).
- Great protective point in pregnancy.

SP13   **Fu She - Bowel Abode**

- Linked to the completion of the digestive process (strong connection with Earth - Tai Yin).

SP 15   **Da Heng - Great Horizontal**

- Hinge point between the upper and lower region (along with ST25 and other points around the sides of the navel).

LV 14   **Qi Men - Cycle Gate**

- Completion.
- Great point to contact the Heart in depth.
- Opens in depth.
- Beginning and end.
- When a person is about to complete something, because this completion allows something else to start.

KD 9	Kidney
SP 12]	
SP 13]	Spleen - Jing / Post-Heaven (Blood)
SP 15]	
SP 16]	
LV 14	Liver – distribution
Heart	Converges at the centre of the chest
CV 22	To bring energy to the head (self-awareness)
CV 23	Window of Heaven
Head / Eyes	Middle of the forehead

Memorisation by the brain of life experiences.

Understanding and overcoming conflict (Heart-Kidney).

This process starts at the Kidneys (KD 9) using its deep energy, to gain experience (Heart) through PC6.

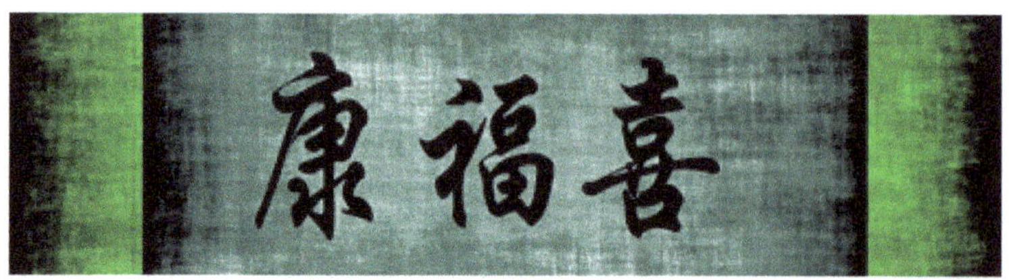

WEI MAI CONSTITUTION

PHYSICAL

- Elegant, beautiful, harmonious, lovely oval face.

- Movements are at times nervous and sometimes a bit artificial.

PSYCHOLOGICAL

- Sensory, and sensitive to the external environment (noise, smells, climatic factors, etc.).

YANG WEI

- Angers easily.
- Finds it difficult to keep to rules.
- Chameleon-like, lacking a clear self-identity, always chasing fashions, moods, trends.
- Tends to easily lose the way, not centred.
- Meteoropathic
- No self-control

YIN WEI

- Hypochondriacs; do not know how to distance themselves and keep the right distance from their feelings and problems, and give them excessive attention.
- Unable to laugh at themselves.
- Introverted, keeps everything inside. Great interior life but not shared with the outside world.

APPLICATIONS

All disorders related to the transition phases of life:

JUVENILE ACNE

- Yang Wei.
- Lung (Connection with the skin).
- GB29 - specific point of transition to adolescence.
- Release points should be checked.

GROWING PAINS DUE TO BONE ELONGATION

Occurs mainly with knee pain.

- Wei Mai.

- Specific points to treat bones (eg. BL11) and local points.

MENARCHE (first menstrual cycle)

Difficulty in starting, stabilizing and regulating the menstrual cycle.

- GB29.

- Chong Mai, Ren Mai (related to Uterus and Blood).

- Spleen (related to Blood).

MENOPAUSE

- Wei Mai.

- Yin in general.

- Kidneys in particular.

- Channels linked to these specific disorders.

E.g: Hot flushes: Kidney and Liver Yin.

        Osteoporosis: Kidney, specific points of the bones and tonification of the blood
        (which nourishes the bones).

AGEING

See below.

PREPARING FOR DEATH

Terminally ill and/or people who feel death is near and who are afraid of dying.

YANG WEI DISORDERS

Linked to symptoms that change and move:

- Pains that move, or come and go.

- Alternating hot and cold.

- Shivers with the sensation of having a fever which is non-existent.

- Cyclothymia (mood swings).

- Manic depression.

- Meteoropathy.

- Dyslexia (non-connection between the two hemispheres).

- Headache radiating from the nape of the neck to the eyes (the Yang Wei path from GB20 going up over the head to the face).

<u>YIN WEI DISORDERS</u>

<u>Connected to Kidney Jing that penetrates the Heart but is not distributed (the 'keeping things inside'):</u>

- <u>Tai Yin Level</u> (SP15 and SP16):

    Slight pain like pins in the heart; intercostal pains, on the sides and abdomen; 'helmet' headache and neck stiffness.

- <u>Jue Yin Level</u> (LV14):

    Severe pain in the heart.

- <u>Shao Yin Level</u> (BL22 and CV23):

    Stabbing pain in the heart, continuous headache (also involves the brain).

<u>Associated with aging:</u>
- Premature aging.
- Physical disorders of old age (osteoporosis, menopause, impotence, etc.).

<u>ANTI-AGING TREATMENT</u>

Both physical and psychological:
- Confluent point of Yin Wei (PC6).
- Confluent point of Yin Qiao (KD6).
- Yin Wei pathway (in particular KD9, SP12, SP13, SP15, SP16, LV14, Heart area, CV22).
- BL1 (Start point of Yin Qiao vessel).

Advise patient to do specific exercises and take regular exercise, etc.

<u>QIAO MAI</u>   Springing Vessels

- Dealing with the outside world, linked to the present moment.

- Self-awareness in relation to the external environment in the present moment.

- Closely connected to the joints, which allow us to move (the ability to move harmoniously).

- To move in the world (along with the Wei).
  While the Wei connect the phases of life in a temporal space, and time, the Qiao are related to the present moment, and to space.

- Strongly connected to trauma, when one remains anchored to a moment or an experience in life.

- Ability to observe, to rise up and see beyond, to see better, both the world (Yang Qiao) and oneself (Yin Qiao), and therefore, to accept things for what they are.

- Start from the feet (roots that sustain the upright position) and finishes at the eyes (to see into the distance).

- The ability to stand upright gives a quality of movement and therefore also a fragility, an instability.

- Accepting the world and themselves makes it possible for changes to take place.

- Encapsulate the Yin-Yang (connected with Du Mai and Ren Mai - Sea of Yin and Sea of Yang).

- Related to structural and constitutional problems, not linked to hereditary but related to the behavioural habits up to the present moment.

- Connected to rhythms in general and in particular to the sleep-wake cycle.

- The Start points are located in the heels (BL62 and KD6).

  The inside part of the foot is arc-shaped, suitable for weight bearing (structure - Yin Qiao) and the outside part is linear which allows movement (Yang Qiao).

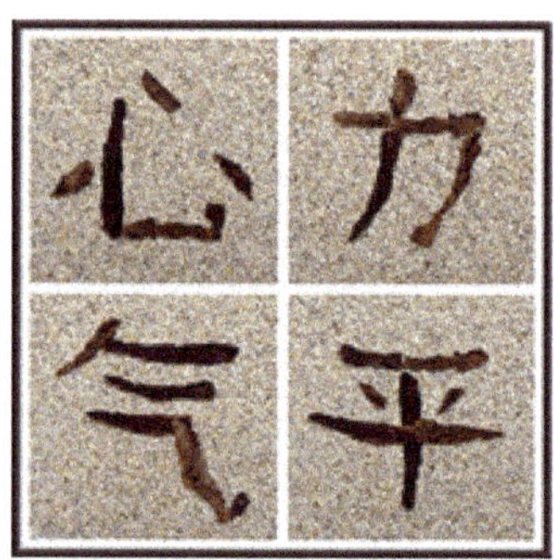

YANG QIAO

Starts at BL62, goes to BL61 and then continues straight along the outside of the leg up to GB29 and then to SI10, LI15, LI16 (from here a branch reaches GB20), ST9, ST4, ST3, ST1 and ends at BL1.

Movement in the present.
To enter into contact with the outside world.

- Joint mobility
- Harmony of movement

Disorders: convulsions, epilepsy, etc.

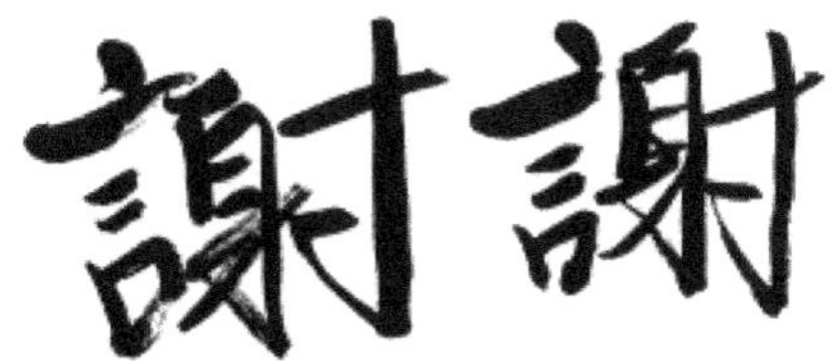

YIN QIAO

Starts at KD2, goes to KD6 and KD8 and then continues along the inside of the leg and enters deep into the side of the abdomen to resurface at ST12; from here it goes to ST9 and ends at BL1.

Awareness in the present.
Process life experiences.

- To look inwards (meditation, consciousness, awareness, etc.) in order to evolve.

Pathologies: stiffness, rigidity (physical and mental).

QIAO MAI CONSTITUTION

<u>PHYSICAL</u>

- Slender people with harmonious, elegant and light gait.
- Elongated neck, outstretched to the sky, almost walking on tiptoe.
- Fine ankles.
- Joint mobility, flexibility.

<u>Pathological:</u>

- Rigid posture.
- Muscle tension (back and femoral quadriceps).
- Joint stiffness (refusal to deal with a situation that needs to be resolved, lack of solidity).
- No roots.

<u>PSYCHOLOGICAL</u>

- Curious, careful, profound people, interested in what lies behind the facade, to experience the world (Yang Qiao).
- Great capacity of introspection (Yin Qiao).
- Depth of character.

<u>Pathological:</u>

Difficulty in accepting:

- themselves:
    - Physical block.
    - Mental rigidity (manic behaviour).
    - Not wanting to breastfeed (the new mother).

- the world:
    - Rejection of the world and/or an urgent need to change it.
    - Hyperactivity (inability to stand still, to stay in the present), with nervous movements
    - Insomnia (mental hyperactivity).

- Internal Wind (muscle tremors, epilepsy, etc.).

- Hypertension, hyperthyroidism.

- Depression, as in low self-esteem that can lead to:

    - weakness in the medial leg;

    - lack of desire to do things;

    - accumulation of Phlegm with stagnation of Dampness due to lack of movement (initially in the limbs and then moving to the internal organs).

- Difficulty in adjusting to new roles and tasks.

- Lack of balance between materiality (Earth) and spirituality (Heaven).

- Pain that occurs simultaneously in multiple zones.

- Disorders relating to the lack of regular habits (sleep, eating, work, shifts ect)

- Lack of 'timing' (including sexual).

- Hypersomnia.

- Digestive problems (Kidney Yang (Fire) that is not activated - KD2), also related to the inability to 'digest' the experiences of life.

YANG QIAO DISORDERS

- Paralysis (inability to physically move in the present), due to:

    - trauma;

    - paraplegia;

    - loss of sense organs (aphonia, deafness etc.).

- Joint problems.

- Convulsions, epilepsy (disharmonious movement).

- Insomnia (the Yang does not yield to the Yin).

- Heat in the skin (Yang remains on the surface - eg. Acne, etc.).

<u>Treatment of the Qiao for joint problems not related to climatic factors</u>

- Opening Point + Qiao Mai vessel.
- Joint mobilization from top to bottom:

> - forehead line / eye line / jaw line;
>
> - neck line, clavicle, scapula and shoulders;
>
> - shoulder / elbow / wrist / finger joints;
>
> - diaphragm / navel / pelvis;
>
> - hip / knee / ankle / toe joints

Work each line: apply pressure on the points that are found there and mobilize the joints.

<u>CONNECTION BETWEEN QIAO MAI AND BACK SHU POINTS</u>

Back Shu =   Basic life conflict management (desire)

Qiao =   Moderate desire, accepting oneself (Yin Qiao - Kidney - KD6) and the world (Yang Qiao - Lung – BL62)

Points =   BL1 related to: - Qiao Mai
                            - Back Shu points

BL11 - BL12 related to Wind (change)

<u>THE ANKLES</u>

Strongly connected to being rooted to the Earth.
"A wise man breathes from his heels."
The centre of the ankle is the place where energy rises to the brain (BL1).
The rigidity of the ankles affects all the other joints.
Mobilizing the neck loosens the limbs and vice versa.

SPECIFIC POINTS OF YANG QIAO

BL62   **Shen Mai - Extending Vessel**

- The Mai that makes us extend.

- Effective point for paralysis.

RELATE TO THE WORLD:

<u>Joints</u>

GB 34 -   knee

GB 29 -   hip

SI 10 -   shoulder

ST 9 -   neck

<u>Sense Organs</u>

ST 3   -   mouth

ST 1   -   eyes

ST 6 - 7 -   ears

ST 8   -   brain

GB 34   **Yang Lin Quan - Yang Mound Spring**

Effective point for all joints.

SPECIFIC POINTS OF YIN QIAO

KD 2   **Ran Gu - Blazing Valley**

(Jing) Spring point of the 5 Transport points, corresponding to the Fire phase.

- Activates the Kidney Yang (Fire) to aid digestion, both physical and of life experiences.

- Burning, 'purifies' to go beyond the experience.

KD 6   Zhao Hai - Shining Sea

Intersection point that opens with the Yin Springing Vessel (Yin Qiao Mai).

- See things for what they are.

- Acceptance (of self and of experience) that, if it happens, a situation of trust develops (KD8).

KD 8   Jiao Xin - Intersection Reach

(Xi) Cleft point of Yin Qiao Mai.

After KD8 the channel goes into the interior to reappear at ST12.

Jiao Xin = to trust

Purifies the Lower Burner

ST 12   Que Pen - Empty Basin

Que = empty, defective

Pen = basin, cup, bowl

Great point of convergence:
- Stomach channel
- All Yang channels (except BL)
- Tendino-Muscular of ST and GB
- Divergent of LI, ST, SP, SI, TB
- Upper Meeting point of Divergent LI - TB

Very important point to eliminate post-natal pathological factors.

ST 9   Ren Ying - Man's Prognosis

Ren = man

Ying = accept, receive, predict, compute

Window of Heaven point.

- Encourages the ascent of Qi to the head.

- "Acceptance" point of cosmic Qi (man's acceptance of his destiny, to be active in the world).

BL 1   **Jing Ming - Bright Eyes**

Union of the Sun and the Moon.

- The dual point closest to the ability to see things in a profound manner (at the centre, Yin Tang, the third eye representing unity)

- Connects the Yin Qiao to the world (through BL1 it is memorized, passed to the brain and to GB20, which represents change). To change through experience.

<u>WINDOWS OF HEAVEN</u>

Treating these points manually is useful when working on the Extraordinary Vessels in order to encourage the ascent or descent of energy.

The six main points are arranged along two lines with three points on each.

Encourages communication between the lower and upper regions and vice versa, and they are used when there is an accumulation/stagnation of energy in the head or in the rest of the body.

In particular:

BL10   Promotes the descent of energy from the head.

ST 9   Promotes the ascent of energy to the head.

ST 9   "Man's Prognosis" – the point where the cosmic Qi enters the human body.

Top Line	SI17	Tian Rong	Celestial Countenance
	TB16	Tian You	Celestial Window
	BL10	Tian Zhu	Celestial Pillar
Bottom Line	ST9	Ren Yin	Man's Prognosis
	LI18	Fu Tu	Protuberance Assistant
	SI16	Tian Chuang	Celestial Window

<u>Summary of the Extraordinary Vessels</u>

FIRST CYCLE 7-8 YEARS

Ancestral	<u>Chong Mai</u>	Trauma in uterus and/or at birth <u>Lack of vital thrust</u>
Birth	<u>Ren Mai</u>	Unity Yin: attachment (1-2 years old) Yang: <u>Lack of nourishment</u>
Separation	<u>Du Mai</u>	individuality, separation (2-3 years) <u>Lack of separation</u>
	<u>Dai Mai</u>	Connection

THE FLOW OF LIFE

Main events in life:	<u>Time</u>: Yang Wei - life choices
	<u>Space</u>: Yin Wei - the distribution of Jing
	Menopause and andropause
	<u>Failure to accept change</u>
Acceptance of the present world:	Self = Yin Qiao
	The world = Yang Qiao
	Physical or psychological trauma
	<u>Failure to accept oneself and the world</u>

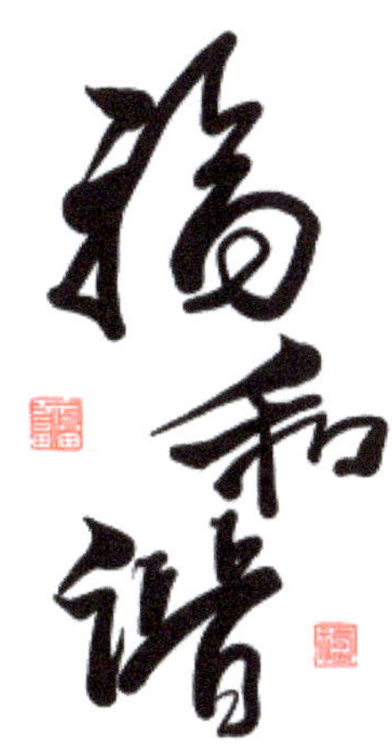

<u>KEYWORDS</u>

<u>CHONG MAI</u>   TRANSFORMATION, CHANGE

<u>DU MAI</u>   ASSERTIVENESS, EVOLUTION

<u>REN MAI</u>   CAREGIVING, RESPONSIBILITY, TAKING CARE OF ONESELF

<u>DAI MAI</u>   COHESION, UNION

<u>WEI MAI</u>   CONNECTION
   <u>YIN:</u>   Connection to internal space, distribution of Kidney Jing
   <u>YANG:</u>   Connection to external space

<u>QIAO MAI</u>   ACCEPTANCE
   <u>YIN:</u>   Acceptance of oneself
   <u>YANG:</u>   Acceptance of the world

The Wei vessels support the Qiao vessels and vice versa.

WAYS OF TREATING THE EXTRAORDINARY VESSELS

Since treatment of these vessels means dealing with far denser and deeper flowing energies, manual treatment should be gentle, and movements slow.

CREATION AND SUPPORT

The possibility to recreate the functions of the Extraordinary Vessel.

- Opening point + vessel pathway (branches) + specific points

Where there is no clear pathological manifestation, but the person is going through a particularly difficult or worrying period.
Treatment offers help and support during this period, increasing the person's capacity to move forward in her life.

REGULATION

Regulates energy.

- Opening point + coupled points + vessel pathway

DEFENCE

When, in a particular moment in life, the energy of the Extraordinary Vessels produces a pathological situation.

- Opening point + Release point + points or sensitive areas on the vessel pathway + related Principle Meridians.

In a particularly arduous or difficult moment in life, and where there is a pathological manifestation that prevents a person from moving forward in their life.

CHONG MAI – PENETRATING VESSEL

CONSTITUTION - DEFICIT

PHYSICAL

- Prevalence of the pelvis over the chest.
- Stocky, overweight.
- Skin disorders (seborrhea, acne, cellulite, etc.).
- Hypertrichosis (hairs are associated with a surplus of blood).
- Lumbago, facet lock (= difficulty to change).

PSYCHOLOGICAL

- Difficulties facing change.
- Habitual (eating habits, roles, etc.).
- Mental rigidity, fixed ideas, traditions, lack of interest for things that change, old before one's time.

DISORDERS

Linked to Blood.
- Endocrine system.
- Menstrual cycle, pregnancy, menopause, etc.
- Hair (surplus of blood).
- Skin (acne, etc.).

1st Branch - KD11 to KD22   Middle Burner – Lower Burner

Digestive, urinary, genital, gynaecological, Rebel Qi, abdominal contractions.

2nd Branch - KD22 to KD27 - CV22 - CV 23   Upper Burner

Cardiovascular, respiratory, cardiac (constitutional).

3rd Branch - Disorders connected to Du Mai

Constitutional Yang deficiency (the Chong Mai did not adequately support the Du Mai).

Down syndrome, mental retardation, contraction, retarded foetus.

Degeneration of the spinal column (osteoporosis – bones not nourished by Blood).

4th Branch

Arterial circulation, aneurysm, hypertension, blood stasis (also affecting venous return).

5th Branch -   KD11 - KD6

Linked to Kidney (constitutional bone, postural, sexual problems).

REN MAI - CONCEPTION VESSEL

CONSTITUTION

PHYSICAL

- Well rooted.

- Bent forward (by the weight of life).

PSYCHOLOGICAL

- Caring

- Independence.

- Ability to take responsibility for one's own life.

DISORDERS

Yin pathology linked to:

- Rootedness

- Solidity

- Conception

- Sexual disorders

- Gynaecological

Gynaecology:

- Menstruation

- Fertility

- Menopause

- Pregnancy

- Childbirth

- Uterus

- Blood

- Tumours

- Hernia

- Fibroids (accumulation of Dampness that generates Heat)

- Asthma, chest tightness, rapid heartbeat, anxiety (Lung has difficulty lowering Qi to the Kidneys – thoracic tract)

<u>When to treat Ren Mai:</u>

- Yin deficiency (and Yang).

  Convalescence, trauma, shock, psychological exhaustion.

- Physical Form.

  Weight loss, obesity, diet and digestive problems, swollen lips and gums (face branch).

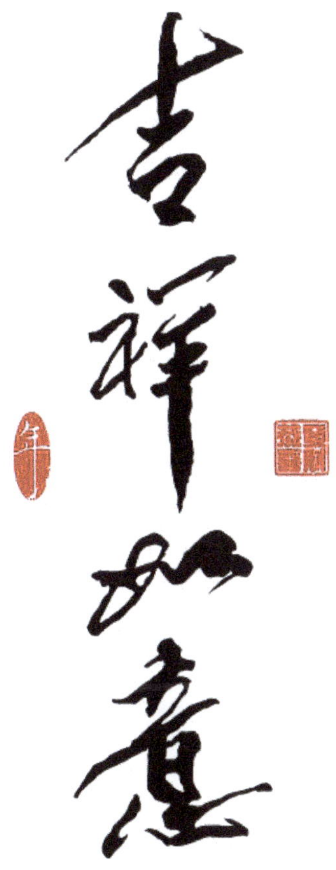

DU MAI- GOVERNING VESSEL

CONSTITUTION

<u>PHYSICAL</u>

- Charismatic
- Well-developed paravertebral muscles.

<u>PSYCHOLOGICAL</u>

- Authoritative
- Control.
- Determination.

<u>DISORDERS</u>

Excess:

- Rigidity of the spinal column
- Interior Wind = epilepsy, Yang insanity (omnipotence, delirium)
- External Wind = fever, runny nose, sensation of head bursting
- Yang that rises too high = stiffness, neck pain, headaches

Deficit:

- Yang deficiency = cold, lower back pain, cold knees, asthenia.
- Incontinence
- Sterility, cold sperm
- Haemorrhoids
- Lack of Jing in the brain = confusion, amnesia, impaired concentration

<u>DAI MAI- GIRDLING VESSEL</u>

CONSTITUTION

<u>PHYSICAL</u>

- Sense of strength
- Cohesion
- Flexible waist
- Top part of body feels hot, lower part feels solid

Disorders:

- Body 'cut in two'
- Top part - very hot
- Lower part - very soft and cold

<u>PSYCHOLOGICAL</u>

- Resolute, determined
- Sense of direction
- Positive criticism
- Well equipped

Disorders:

- Missing, lost
- Incoherent
- Indecisive
- Hypercritical, intolerant
- Resentful, bitter

<u>DISORDERS</u>

- Communication between high-low.
- Strong bond with Spleen and Liver
- Pathologies relating to Dampness (SP) and stasis (LV).

<u>Damp-Cold:</u>

- Dysentery, undigested food
- Fibroids
- Impotence
- Sterility

If the Heat remains in the lower region:

- Genital and urinary inflammation
- Prostatitis
- Cystitis
- Priapism (prolonged erection)

If the Heat rises:

- Anxiety, panic
- Irritability

WEI MAI – LINKING VESSELS

CONSTITUTION

<u>PHYSICAL</u>

- Elegant, beautiful, harmonious
- Nervous
- Artificial

<u>PSYCHOLOGICAL</u>

- Sensorial, sensitive
- Moody
- Changeable
- Meteor sensitive

Yang Wei = no self-control

Yin Wei = keeps everything inside

<u>DISORDERS</u>

Connection between the stages of life

- Acne in adolescence

- Pain caused by the lengthening growth of bones

- Menstrual disorders

- Menopausal disorders

- Aging

- Death

<u>YIN WEI</u>

Connects the Yin areas to each other and to the Yang.

If the Yin remains trapped deep down (blood is blocked within):

- Pains in the heart that are more painful the deeper the level of the Yin in which the blood is trapped:

  - Tai Yin: slight pains, intercostal, sides, helmet headache, stiff neck

  - Jue Yin: very strong and more localized pain

  - Shao Yin: continuous headaches

<u>YANG WEI</u>

Connects the Yang with the Yin.

If the Yang remains on the exterior the distinction between one's own space and that of the exterior is lost:

- Mood swings (cyclothymia)

- Manic depression

- Meteoropathy

- Volatility

QIAO MAI- SPRINGING VESSELS

CONSTITUTION

<u>PHYSICAL</u>

- Long-limbed

- Elongated neck

- Light (almost walking on tiptoe)

- Elegant

- Thin ankles

<u>PSYCHOLOGICAL</u>

- Curious

- Careful

- Eager to know what lies beyond mere appearances.

- Introspective

<u>DISORDERS</u>

Sleep-wake rhythm

- Yin Qiao = insomnia

- Yang Qiao = hypersomnia

<u>YIN QIAO</u>

Linked to Kidneys.

- Digestive disorders (physical and psychological - KD2)

- Structural defects, not constitutional (infantile scoliosis)

- Joint problems

<u>YANG QIAO</u>

- Blocked joints, paralysis

- Blocked joints caused by unresolved trauma

- Convulsions, epilepsy

- Heat in the skin (acne, etc.)

<u>To free the shoulders, chest, to encourage circulation</u>: important points GB 22 -SP 21

<u>To lower blood pressure:</u> SP 21 (same level as CV15)

<u>Menstrual problems</u>: most problems are caused by blood deficiency or blood stagnation:

BLOOD STAGNATION
Pains before the onset of menstruation caused by a deficiency or a stasis of blood:
LV + Dai Mai + Chong Mai

BLOOD DEFICIENCY
Pain during menstruation and at the end of cycle:
SP + Chong Mai

LONG MENSTRUATION
Spleen - SP4 - BL11 - LV12 - ST30 - SP12
If Kidney involved also treat sacral foramina points.

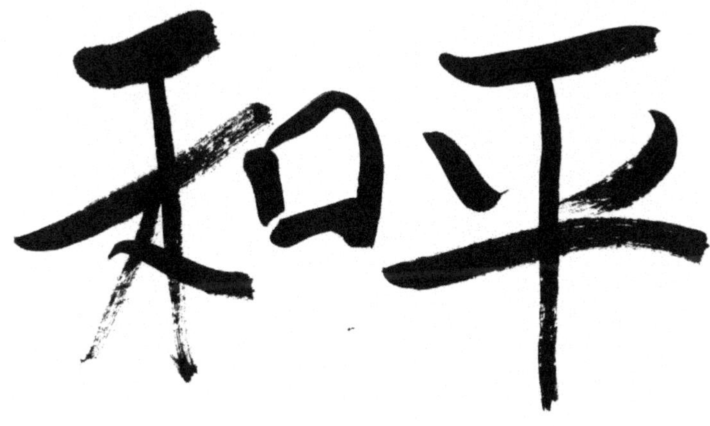

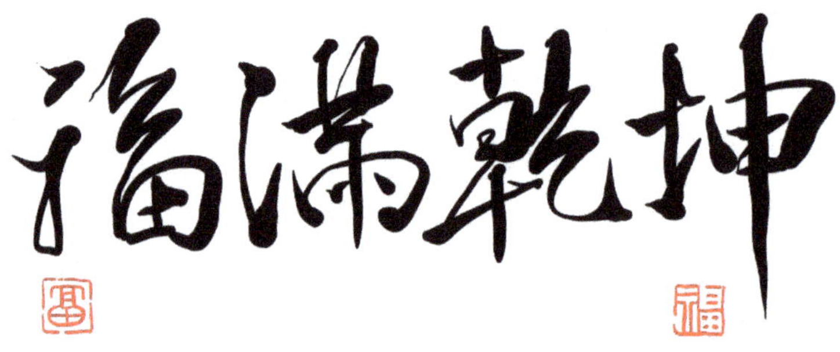

BIBLIOGRAPHY

D.M. Connelly 'Traditional Acupuncture: The Law of the five elements'.
F. Bottalo 'Fondamenti di Medicina Tradizionale Cinese'(Foundations of TCM).
F. Bottalo 'Diagnosi Shiatsu' (Shiatsu Diagnosis).
F. Bottalo 'Manuale di Shiatsu' (Shiatsu Manual).
F. Bottalo 'Manuale di Qi Shu' (Qi Shu Manual).
A. Gulì 'Le acque lunari – La medicina cinese e la donna' (Woman in TCM).
Lu Tzu 'The Mystery of the Golden Flower'.
G. Maciocia 'The Foundations of Chinese Medicine'.
Huang Ti 'Nei Ching Su Wen: The Yellow Emperor's Classic on Internal Medicine'.
L.V. Arena 'Nei-Ching - I fondamenti della Medicina Tradizionale Cinese'.
W. Ohashi 'Eastern Diagnosis'.
W. Ohashi 'Shiatsu'.
G. Allasia 'Self-Shiatsu'.
S. Masunaga 'Zen Shiatsu'.
S. Masunaga 'Zen imaging'.
Masunaga S. & W. Ohashi 'Zen Shiatsu'.
P. Lundberg 'The illustrated manual of Shiatsu'.
C. Beresford-Cooke 'Shiatsu Theory and Practice'.
J. Schatz, C. Larre, Rochat E. De La Vallee 'Elements of Traditional Chinese Medicine'.
T.J. Kaptchuk 'Chinese Medicine, foundations and method'.
T. Namikoshi 'Shiatsu'.
T. Namikoshi 'The Complete Book of Shiatsu'.
Lao Tzu 'Tao Te Ching'.
'I Ching, the Book of Changes'.

Atlas of Acopuncture.

Contents   *329*

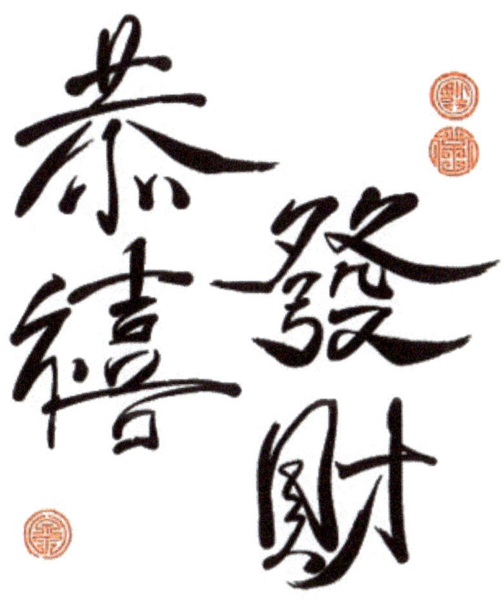

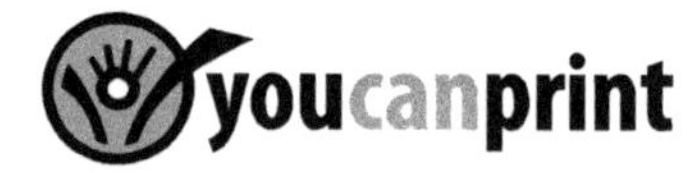

Printed in the month May 2016
behalf of Youcanprint *Self - Publishing*